7 Ke
Your Cholesterol Level

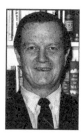

About the Author

Dr. Bruce Miller's postgraduate studies at New York University included clinical, nutrition oriented research which focused on nutrition problems of the elderly.

Dr. Miller is a member of the Linus Pauling Institute of Science Medicine, a charter member of Dr. Kenneth Cooper's Aerobics Center, a member of the International Academy of Preventive Medicine, International College of Applied Nutrition, founder of the Diet Analysis Center, and a consultant to the American Running and Fitness Association.

Dr. Miller is a Certified Nutrition Specialist and a member of the American College of Nutrition. Currently Dr. Miller is the Director of Research for the American Academy of Nutrition. Dr. Miller lives in Dallas with Jody, his wife of more than 40 years.

Published in arrangement with Oak Publications Sdn Bhd.

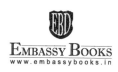

Published in India by :
EMBASSY BOOKS,
120 Great Western Building,
M.C. C. Lane, Kala Ghoda, Fort,
Mumbai - 400 023.
Tel : +9122 22819546 / 32967415
Email : info@embassybooks.in
www.embassybooks.in

ISBN : 978-93-83359-84-4

Key #1

Understand Your
Blood Lipid Profile

❝ What are all of these numbers we are supposed to know?" Ann exclaimed to her friend while waving a sheet of paper containing her current blood lipids.

"My cholesterol is 5.46 and my doctor says don't worry about it, but then I read in a magazine that 5.46 is high," sighed Ann. "Also, what in the world are triglycerides, LDLs, HDLs and all of that other stuff?" Ann shook her head in worry. "I know I am supposed to increase fiber in my diet; I wonder if lettuce is high fiber?" Ann gave an angry grimace, "I sometimes just feel like giving up; there is so much confusion."

Ann is right; there is lot of confusion. I will explain the "blood lipid profile" values, and give you reasonable ways to decrease your chances of a heart attack. Most people can cut their risk of heart attack by 50 percent if they are willing to make a few simple changes in their lifestyles. The evidence is overwhelming!

By the way, Ann, who has a cholesterol reading of 5.46 is 70 years old, walks three miles a day, has never smoked, is at her exact weight and is taking two courses at a local university. She should probably be more worried about her college grades than her cholesterol.

Are you confused by all of the lipid (blood fat) terms such as HDL, LDL, Total cholesterol, ratio of Total cholesterol to HDL, saturated and mono-unsaturated fats, etc? We are going to make all the healthy terms and numbers make sense, so you will know the importance to you and your heart's health. Some people get so confused and frustrated that they throw up their hands in disgust and head for the local fast food (grease pit) establishment for a quick coronary "lube" job. Don't give up! Keep reading!

MAKING SENSE OF CHOLESTEROL

Measuring Cholesterol
In the United States, cholesterol is measured in milligrams per deciliter (mg/dL). In some countries it is measured in millimols per liter (mmol/L). Following are the conversion formulas:

Cholesterol Conversion
mg/dL of cholesterol x 0.02586 = mmol/L
mmol/L of cholesterol x 38.67 = mg/dL

Triglyceride Number Conversion
mg/dL of triglyceride x 0.01129 = mmol/L
mmol/L of triglyceride x 88.496 = mg/dL

All cholesterol measurements in this book refer to mmol/L.

Cholesterol and Lipoproteins

Cholesterol is a fat-like substance that circulates in your blood and tissues. The liver produces about 1,000 milligrams of cholesterol a day. About 150 to 250 milligrams of cholesterol come from what you eat daily, mainly from animal sources. Vegetables, fruits and grains contain no cholesterol.

Cholesterol and other fats can't dissolve in the blood – just like oil and water, the two do not mix. They have to be transported to and from the cells by special carriers called lipoproteins. These lipoproteins are made of fat (lipid) on the inside and protein on the outside. Two kinds of lipoproteins carry cholesterol throughout your body. It is important to have healthy levels of both.

Lipoproteins are either high-density or low-density, based on how much protein and fat they have. The lower the density of the lipoprotein, the more fat it contains. These proteins act like trucks, picking up the cholesterol and transporting it to different parts of the body.

There are two major types of lipoprotein that transport cholesterol through your blood circulatory system – low-density lipoprotein (LDL) and high-density lipoprotein (HDL).

We need a balance bewtween the "good" HDL cholesterol and the "bad" LDL cholesterol for optimal health.

HDL – The Good Side of Cholesterol

Cholesterol builds and repairs cells. Cholesterol is part

of all cell membranes: Liver, skin, brain cells, nerve tissue and intestines. Cholesterol is also part of the myelin sheath that surrounds and protects nerves, and it is used to make vitamin D.

It is used to produce sex hormones like estrogen and testosterone. Cholesterol participates in the formation of bile acids in the liver to help in digestion. A large amount of cholesterol is found in the brain and nerve tissue.

HDL is the life-saving lipoprotein and considered a good cholesterol. HDL contains more protein than cholesterol or fat. HDL cholesterol helps prevent harmful build-up of cholesterol in your arteries by carrying it back to the liver for disposal. In so doing, it reduces cholesterol, and lessens the chance of being deposited in the arteries.

A high level of HDL cholesterol may lower your chances of developing heart attack or stroke.

Besides picking up excess cholesterol and bringing it back to the liver for disposal, HDL also:

- Acts as an antioxidant which helps neutralize free radicals that contribute to atherosclerosis

- Is an anti-inflammatory (like aspirin) and can decrease the inflammation linked with the atherosclerotic process

- Lessens the ability of the blood to form clots, thus reducing the risk of heart attack or stroke

LDL Cholesterol: The Dark Side

LDL is loaded with cholesterol and is the major carrier of cholesterol from the liver to the rest of the body. It is the chief cholesterol carrier in the blood, carrying approximately 70 percent of all the blood cholesterol around the network of arteries.

Unlike HDL, LDL is not directly manufactured in the liver. Instead, a different type of lipoprotein is first produced by the liver, the parent molecule called Very Low Density Protein (VLDL). After circulating around the bloodstream, VLDL loses much of its fat (triglyceride) cache to various bodily cells to become LDL.

LDL is designed to take cholesterol to cells that require some cholesterol to maintain proper functioning of the body. Typically, the LDL is taken into the cell and broken down, and then the cholesterol is used to make membranes or hormones.

When cholesterol levels are excessive, LDL deposits cholesterol onto the arteries causing the damage. For this reason, LDL is often referred to as "bad" cholesterol.

LDL cholesterol carries mostly fat and only a small amount of protein from the liver to other parts of the body. We know that if LDL levels rise too high, cholesterol can pile up in the arteries' inner wall and atherosclerosis begins with the narrowing of the large arteries that supply blood to the heart.

Oxidized LDL: The True Culprit

This is not the whole story. New research is showing

that oxidized LDL (OXLDL) is the true culprit of heart disease.

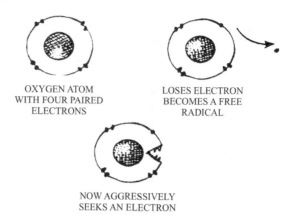

OXYGEN ATOM
WITH FOUR PAIRED
ELECTRONS

LOSES ELECTRON
BECOMES A FREE
RADICAL

NOW AGGRESSIVELY
SEEKS AN ELECTRON

Free radicals in action

A single free radical starts a chain reaction and oxidizes many LDL molecules. It's much like a row of toppling dominoes. A free radical sticks to an LDL particle, which passes it to another LDL molecule and so on.

Each LDL particle in turn becomes oxidized. The oxidized LDL has properties totally different from normal LDL. It seems charged with artery-clogging power, a deadly particle to our arteries. Let's take a look at how OXLDL does its dirty work.

Oxidized LDL (OXLDL) appears to be the main player in heart disease. A three-stage attack is waged in order to damage arteries and trigger atherosclerosis. The news from researchers is that oxidized LDL is not only present in all three stages but it actually speeds up atherosclerosis development.

Stage One

Plaque buildup begins when the inner lining of a coronary artery is damaged by OXLDL. Cells lining the artery fit tightly together. OXLDL attacks and changes the appearance and functions of these cells; they now fit loosely. "Normal" LDL does not cause this damage.

Stage Two

The macrophage is one of the main "garbage disposal" cells of the body. It will eat foreign invaders and cell wastes. These are "digested" by the macrophages and rendered harmless.

The macrophages ignore normal LDL but recognize OXLDL as foreign particles and eat them. Here is the big problem. The macrophages cannot digest the OXLDL, so this fat accumulates and the macrophages become obese. When this happens and the macrophages become fat enough, they migrate to your artery wall through the loosened cells lining the wall. Once in the artery wall, the macrophage is now called a foam cell. This cell migration causes the artery wall to bulge out into the lumen (inner lining) which reduces the size of the artery opening. Thus, potentially deadly plaque has begun to grow.

Stage Three

Foam cells continue to grow and build artery-clogging plaque through their appetite for fat – mostly OXLDL. To worsen the situation, as they eat and grow, they produce even more free radicals.

THE BLOOD LIPID PROFILE TEST

Managing your cholesterol is part of a lifelong commitment to reduce your risk of cardiovascular disease. It is important therefore to schedule with your doctor a blood test that will provide you with your cholesterol numbers before beginning any program for lowering it.

Before the Test

It is best to fast for 12 hours before your test if you want an accurate picture of your blood lipid profile as triglycerides and LDL are influenced by what you eat. Also limit your physical activity before the test.

You can drink water in the time leading up to the test, but avoid coffee, tea and other beverages. Talk to your doctor about any other special requirements. Some medications, such as birth control pills, can increase your cholesterol levels.

The National Cholesterol Education Program (NCEP) Panel, an expert group of doctors and scientists affiliated with the National Institute of Health, recommends that all people older than age 20 have a fasting blood test called a lipoprotein profile every five years as well as for children in families with cardiovascular risk factors.

Periodic lipid testing will determine whether you have met your goals or need more intensive treatment. NCEP Guidelines recommend testing every six weeks until lipid goals are met and every four to six months thereafter.

The Test: Blood Sample
Your doctor normally will draw blood for the test from your veins in your arm. The point where he will insert the needle is cleaned with antiseptic and an elastic band is wrapped around your upper arm to restrict blood flow through your vein. This causes the veins to be filled with blood.

Next, he gently inserts a needle into the vein. The blood collects into an airtight vial or tube attached to the needle. The elastic band is removed from your arm to restore circulation, and blood continues to flow into the vial. Once enough blood is collected, the needle is removed, and the puncture site is covered with a plaster to stop any bleeding or infection.

The entire procedure will likely last a couple of minutes. It is relatively painless. Some people do, however, feel moderate pain when the needle is inserted, while others feel only a tiny pinprick.

The blood sample taken will be sent to a licensed laboratory approved by the National Cholesterol Education Program (NCEP) for analysis.

New Cholesterol Testing Technology
A new type of cholesterol test called a nuclear magnetic resonance (NMR) spectroscopy is now available. This technique can measure the size and number of your LDL and HDL particles.

Researchers now believe that knowing the size and quantity of each type of LDL and HDL particle present in your blood might be a more precise indicator of your risk of heart disease than just measuring the cholesterol in the LDL and HDL lipoproteins. More research is needed to perfect this technique and its usefulness is ongoing.

Who Should Go for a Cholesterol Test?

High blood cholesterol itself does not cause any symptoms; so many people are unaware of their cholesterol level. Cholesterol lowering is important for everyone – the young, the middle age, the elderly and people with or without heart disease.

Men and women 20 years and older should undergo cholesterol screening every five years. Women before menopause have levels that are lower than men of the same age. After menopause, a women's LDL level goes up, and so her risk for heart disease increases. For both men and women, heart disease is the number one cause of death.

Pregnant women should wait at least six weeks after giving birth to have their cholesterol measured; as cholesterol is often high during pregnancy.

What Does a Blood Lipid Profile Include?

A complete blood lipid profile is an analysis of the fats in your blood. They should include the following:

- Total cholesterol (TC)
- LDL – the "bad cholesterol"
- HDL – the "good cholesterol"
- Ratio of TC to HDL
- Triglycerides (TG)

In the future, a test called ApoB (Apolipo-protein) may become a routine test for cholesterol. ApoB is the protein portion of the LDL molecule and testing this protein may be the most accurate estimate or marker for LDL that is circulating in the blood stream. In the future, instead of just testing for LDL and HDL, you may also need to know your ApoB.

Grim Figures
Cholesterol is one of the risk factors of heart attack and stroke. The statistics are not too good so far as heart disease goes. This year about 1.5 million Americans will have a heart attack. Of these, 550,000 will die. These tragic figures can be greatly improved based on current knowledge. How?

Listen to this from the American Heart Association: "A major reduction in both heart attack and heart death can be achieved only by prevention of hearts attacks, not from the treatment of established disease. Almost half of all heart attack deaths occur with the first heart attack and before treatment can be started. Therefore, prevention is a must."

GUIDELINES TO YOUR LIPID PROFILE

I have put together a complete graphical lipid profile guideline for your easy reference. It is important that you keep your lipids in the normal range. If your number is above 3.36, take aggressive steps to lower it by following the recommendations outlined in my book.

Cholesterol Profile

LDL: The Bad Cholesterol

Less than 2.56	Optimal
2.57 - 3.36	Near/Above Optimal
Above 3.36 - 4.11	Borderline High
Above 4.11 - 4.99	High
Above 4.99	Very High

Your desirable LDL level is below 3.36.

High-Density Lipoprotein:
The Life-saving Lipoprotein

More than 1.16 for men	Desirable
More than 1.55 for women	Desirable

The desirable level of HDL cholesterol is more than 1.16 for men and more than 1.55 for women.

Total Cholesterol

5.17	Desirable
Above 5.17-6.18	Borderline High
More than 6.18	High

The desirable level of Total cholesterol is less than 5.17.

This is a sum of your blood's cholesterol content. It's possible to measure only Total cholesterol. However, this single test isn't used as much anymore, because knowing only your Total cholesterol level doesn't provide your doctor with much useful information.

Total Cholesterol / HDL Ratio: Best Predictor of Heart Disease

Research has found the ratio of Total cholesterol to HDL to be the best predictor of heart disease. You divide the Total cholesterol by the HDL. This ratio is perhaps more important than Total cholesterol. High Total cholesterol and low HDL cholesterol increases the ratio, and is undesirable. Conversely, high HDL cholesterol and low Total cholesterol lowers the ratio, and is desirable.

4.5 or lower for men	Desirable
4.0 or lower for women	Desirable

The desirable TC/HDL ratio range is 4.5 or less for men and less than 4.0 for women.

The Mystery

The mystery about Total cholesterol has been this: Why do we see heart attacks in people with fairly low Total cholesterol while in others with high cholesterol, no heart attack? Let me give you an example.

	Person A	Person B
Total Cholesterol	6.47	5.17
HDL	1.29	0.52
Ratio	5	10

Person A has a much higher Total cholesterol than person B. It would seem that he is in trouble, right? Actually person B with his "normal" cholesterol number is at a much greater risk for a heart attack than person A.

The major difference is the vitally important ratio. Studies have revealed that the high ratio in people with low Total cholesterol levels is one explanation why a person with low cholesterol will have a heart attack. Person A should get his cholesterol down because that is still a separate risk factor, but risk-wise, he is in better shape as he has a lower ratio than person B.

If your Total cholesterol is above 5.17, be sure to check the ratio. The normal ratio for men is 4.5 or lower, and for women 4.0 or lower. Research tells us that 3.5 is good and below 3.0 is excellent.

Several studies support the fact that if you can get your ratio to between 2.4 and 2.8, you can actually get reversal of heart coronary artery disease.

It is important to remember that even with a favorable ratio; it is still imperative that you get your LDL to less than 2.56 regardless of the HDL value, especially in the presence of other multiple risk factors for coronary artery disease such as genetic pre-disposition, smoking, hypertension, and diabetes. In patients with known coronary artery disease such as a history of bypass surgery, an LDL of less than 2.56 is extremely desirable.

Triglycerides Profile
When you get a blood lipid profile, you will get a number for something called triglycerides. Triglycerides are, for simplification, what we call "fat." When you grab a handful of tummy, love handles, or some other fat storage, you are grabbing triglycerides. Triglycerides are produced in the body from the fats you eat or excess calories coming from alcohol or carbohydrate-rich foods.

Triglycerides come from both animal or plant foods, while cholesterol comes from animal foods only. Triglycerides contain fatty acids while cholesterol does not. Unlike triglycerides, cholesterol does not provide any calories.

High triglycerides is a risk factor to be considered because it is consistently associated with high LDL and low HDL. The mechanism of this association is not well understood, but high triglycerides is considered a heart attack risk factor. An ideal number for triglycerides is below 1.41.

Triglycerides

Less than 1.41	Desirable
Above 1.41 – 2.24	Borderline High
Above 2.24 – 5.63	High
Above 5.63	Very High

DESIRABLE SUMMARY NUMBER LINE UP

Let's do a fast summary of the blood lipid profile we have so far discussed. There are several numbers that must line up correctly. Remember, each is a separate risk factor. The two most significant are the TC/HDL ratio and the Total cholesterol. Compare your numbers you got from your doctor earlier with the lipid blood profile outlined below. If your tests show that your numbers are not in alignment with the desirable lipid lineup, the steps ahead will show you how to improve your numbers.

The Desirable Number Line Up Without Personal History of Heart or Vessel Disease

Total cholesterol	Less than 5.17
HDL cholesterol	More than 1.16 for men
	More than 1.55 for women
LDL cholesterol	Less than 3.36
Triglycerides	Less than 1.41
Total cholesterol/HDL ratio	4.5 or less for men
	4.0 or less for women

Pay attention, because this is crucial. If just one factor in your lipid profile is abnormal, it is a separate risk factor. For optimal coronary protection, all factors must be in good ranges. Dr William Castelli of the famous Framingham Heart Study says you must know four numbers to stay alive: Your Total cholesterol, HDL cholesterol, your triglycerides, and your Social Security number.

"If you keep your Total cholesterol/HDL ratio under 4.5, your LDL cholesterol under 3.36, your triglycerides under 1.41, you exercise, and don't smoke, you will very probably never have a heart attack," says Dr Castelli. Get your numbers checked now by a good laboratory.

THE DANGERS OF EXCESS CHOLESTEROL

Dr Kenneth Cooper aptly says, "A very important part of preventing heart attacks is controlling your cholesterol – not eliminating it all together."

The "cholesterol hypothesis" is no longer a hypothesis. "There is no doubt that abnormal cholesterol levels cause morbidity and mortality and that aggressive treatment saves lives." (*Journal of the American Medical Association* 2001: 285: 2508-2509).

We need to lower cholesterol because it is accepted worldwide as the best indicator of the rate your arteries (and you) are aging. To slow that rate, lower your cholesterol and keep it down. Excess cholesterol causes:

Aging Coronary Arteries

As the artery ages, sludge, gunk, or the scientific word "plaque," deposits in the artery walls. This plaque is mostly cholesterol. It's pretty simple; the higher your cholesterol level, the more rapidly plaque develops in your arteries.

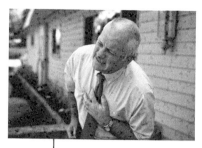

When should you begin to worry? This process can begin with fatty streaks in the artery as young as 11 years of age. If your family has a history of high cholesterol or early death caused by heart attack, have your child's cholesterol checked. This establishes a base line to which you can refer back to in later years.

Plugged Plumbing

Plaque is somewhat like the scale that builds up inside a water pipe. It isn't noticed until the flow of water slows down or the water won't flow at all. A similar event is occurring in your heart's vessels, but you can't handle it as easily as calling a plumber.

As plaque builds, the coronary artery's opening narrows. Because the blood flow is restricted to the heart, you will get shortness of breath on exertion, or even chest pain. Other symptoms include headache, nausea or vomiting, sweating, heartburn or indigestion, and arm pain. Sometimes, one quarter of heart attacks are silent, especially in people with diabetes.

The aging of the coronary arteries and excess cholesterol unused by the body can cause the build-up of plaque on our artery walls, leading to the blockage of one or more arteries resulting in:

- **A Heart Attack (Myocardial Infarction)**

  This occurs when the blood supply to part of the heart muscle itself is severely reduced or blocked. This is usually caused by the buildup of plaque, a process called atherosclerosis. If the blood supply is cut off for more than a few minutes, heart muscle cells suffer permanent injury and die. This can kill or disable someone, depending on how much heart muscle is damaged.

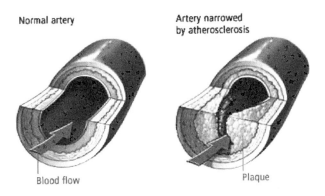

Normal artery

Artery narrowed by atherosclerosis

Blood flow

Plaque

Symptoms of an impending heart attack can be vague and mild. Many people attribute heart attack symptoms to indigestion, heartburn, fatigue or stress, and so discount seeking early medical attention. This can prove fatal for many people.

Bystanders can help save the life of a heart attack victim by cardiopulmonary resuscitation (CPR) which involves breathing for the victim (mouth-to-mouth) and applying external compression to squeeze the heart and force it to pump blood.

- **A Stroke**

  A stroke, sometimes called a "brain attack", is caused by a massive blood clot blocking the flow of blood to the brain or bleeding in the brain. A person's speech, writing, balance, sensation, memory, thinking, attention, and learning are some of the areas that can be affected as a result of suffering a stroke.

HIGHLIGHTS OF THE NEW CHOLESTEROL GUIDELINES BY THE US NATIONAL CHOLESTEROL AND EDUCATION PROGRAM (MAY 2001)

- People with multiple risk factors for heart disease should keep their LDL less than 2.59 and those with LDL of 3.36 or higher should undergo drug therapy and therapeutic lifestyle changes, which include reduced intake of saturated fats and cholesterol, weight reduction and increased physical activity.

- Type 2 diabetics with high cholesterol should be treated more aggressively whether or not clinical coronary disease is present.

- HDL level of less than 1.03 is considered a risk factor for heart disease, as compared to 0.91 recommended in 1993. A HDL of 1.55 or more is considered protective against heart disease.

- Men and women over 20 years should have their Total cholesterol, LDL, HDL and triglycerides tested once every five years.

- People with borderline levels of triglycerides are advised to lose weight and exercise. High triglycerides may warrant medication.

- Adults are advised to lower their LDL level through diet before trying medication.

- Lowering LDL can reduce the short-term risk of heart disease by as much as 40 percent.

- Foods that contain plant stanols and sterols, or are rich in soluble fiber, can boost the diet's LDL-lowering power.

- Hormone Replacement Therapy is not advisable as an alternative to cholesterol-lowering drugs.

Key #2

Eat Heart Healthy Food

There's no denying that a healthy diet is the first line of defense against rising cholesterol. "If you eat a predominantly plant-based diet—with lots of fruits and vegetables plus some fish—you are on the right track to keeping your cholesterol at a healthy level," says Lisa Dorfman, a registered dietitian and spokeswoman for the American Dietetic Association.

High levels of the wrong types of cholesterol can lead to the development of arterial plaque which can increase the risks for heart disease, stroke and other conditions related to the cardiovascular system.

KNOW YOUR FATS

Table 1 illustrates the various types of fats that are available in your diet. Values are expressed as percent of total fats; data are sourced from the Harvard School of Public Health Lipid Laboratory and U.S.D.A publications.

Table 1

Percentage of Specific Types of Fat in Common Oils and Fats*			
Oils	Saturated	Mono-unsaturated	Poly-unsaturated	Trans
Olive	13	72	8	0
Canola	7	58	29	0
Peanut	17	49	32	0
Soybean	16	44	37	0
Palm	50	37	10	0
Corn	13	24	60	0
Sunflower	10	20	66	0
Safflower	9	12	74	0
Coconut	87	6	2	0
Cooking Fats			
Shortening	22	29	29	18
Lard	39	44	11	1
Butter	60	26	5	5
Margarine/Spreads			
70% Soybean Oil, Stick	18	2	29	23
67% Corn & Soybean Oil Spread, Tub	16	27	44	11
48% Soybean Oil Spread, Tub	17	24	49	8
60% Sunflower, Soybean, and Canola Oil Spread, Tub	18	22	54	5

* Values expressed as percent of total fat; data are from analyses at Harvard School of Public Health Lipid Laboratory and U.S.D.A. publications.

THE GOAL

The cholesterol lowering diet's goal is oriented to reduce your Total cholesterol level, improve your ratio of Total cholesterol to HDL and to reduce your risk of heart disease.

The Report of the National Cholesterol Education Program Expert Panel on Detection, Evaluation, and Treatment of High Blood Cholesterol in Adults repeatedly advocate that dietary control is the primary cholesterol-lowering treatment and should be the first line of attack.

The panel also strongly recommends the following:

- We consume less than 200 mg of dietary cholesterol. It also allows up to 35 percent of daily calories from total fat, provided most of it comes from unsaturated fats which do not cause a rise in cholesterol levels.

- Fifty to sixty percent of calories should come from less processed, higher fiber carbohydrates. Intake of high carbohydrates (greater than 60 percent of daily calories) may cause a reduction in HDL cholesterol, although there is no strong evidence to suggest that it affects LDL cholesterol.

In a statement in 2006, the American Heart Association says, "Another major change in the dietary recommendations is a lower goal for saturated fat – from less than 10 percent to less than seven percent – and establishing a goal for trans fatty acids of less than one percent of total calories."

We suggest the following action plan for a healthy heart:

MINIMIZE INTAKE OF SATURATED FATS

Saturated fats have high melting points and are usually solid at room temperature. Eating excessive saturated fats can increase cholesterol in your blood more than consuming cholesterol!

This is what happens: As fat is an unstable molecule, cholesterol helps stabilize the saturated fat molecule. It takes two molecules of cholesterol to stabilize one molecule of saturated fat. Therefore, if you have a diet high in saturated fats, more cholesterol must be available to work with the fat, so your body ends with more cholesterol in your blood.

Good Side of Saturated Fats
Like cholesterol, your body needs saturated fats to function properly. Besides being an energy source, fat is a nutrient used in the production of cell membranes, they enhance the immune system and they help incorporate calcium into your bones.

However, it is when you consume too much saturated fats damaged by heat, oxygen, and unnatural farming practices that becomes harmful to your heart health.

What to Avoid
Here are some ways you can do to lower your saturated fats from your diet by reducing the intake of:

- Dairy fats such as butter, clarified butter, cultured butter, butter/margarine mix.

- Milk homogenized or full cream.

- Hard cheeses, cream cheese, sour cream, ice cream and dressing – avoid using them, especially for your salad dressing.

- Meat fats: Lard, dripping, suet and beef tallow.

- White visible fat on: Beef, mutton, lamb, pork and poultry – trim the skin from chicken and turkey and the fat from beef.

- Processed meat: Luncheon, salami, most sausages, tinned corned beef, fatty mince pies and pates.

- Watch for hidden saturated fats in deep fried foods, fast foods and processed foods.

- Limit your intake of food with gravies and sauces.

- Refined sugars: Do not add to foods.

What is Left?

Good grief, what can you eat? The following is a suggested food plan that you should follow for good health and maximum energy, even if your cholesterol is normal:

- Eat fowl with skin removed.

- If you love desserts, purchase or learn how to make low-fat, high-fiber treats such as oatmeal cookies, fruit crumble or cakes made with whole-wheat flour and unsaturated fats.

- Use olive-oil-based salad dressings. Add sunflower seeds or nuts to salads instead of bacon bits.

- For snacks, instead of choosing high-fat junk food such as French fries or potato chips, have nuts, peanut butter on whole wheat bread, vegetables, fruits, chips or cakes made from brown rice or soy.

- Eat cold water fish such as salmon, cod, sardine, trout, herring and mackerel at least three times a week. They contain omega-3 fatty acid, a good fat. EPA and DHA help disperse saturated fat and helps platelets from getting "sticky" to open up our arteries.

- Use omega-6, another essential fatty acid found in unrefined oils such as olive oil, avocados, flax seeds, almonds, peanuts, borage seed oil, grape seed oil, and evening primrose oil.

- Eat a variety of rainbow colored vegetables and fruits. According to the National Heart, Lung and Blood Institute's Family Heart

Study, participants who ate four or more servings of fruits and vegetables a day had significantly lower levels of LDL cholesterol than those who ate fewer servings. Among the most powerful veggies are the dark green, leafy variety, such as spinach, kale, collard greens and Swiss chard. They contain vitamins, minerals and phytonutrients rich in antioxidants, soluble and insoluble fibers. Go organic whenever possible.

- Do less frying, instead bake, sauté, boil, poach, roast, broil or steam your food.

- Beans and lentils – beware of fat content.

- Oat and oat bran.

- Drink at least eight glasses of clean purified water.

- Avoid using any cooking oil that has been processed or refined. Instead, look for virgin or unrefined oil for your cooking purposes.

- Use fat sparingly. Put less butter on your bread or potato, less salad dressing on your salad and so on.

- Use garlic generously in your cooking.

- Use low-fat or non-fat milk or no-fat yogurt and cheese or cottage cheese.

INCREASE INTAKE OF GOOD FATS

A healthy liver manufactures most of our daily essential cholesterol requirements. Additional cholesterol in the foods we eat (dietary cholesterol) is absorbed in the intestines and elevates blood cholesterol.

Here are some foods that can be of help to reduce dietary cholesterol in your diet:

Monounsaturated Fats (Unrefined)

According to the NCEP, monounsaturated fats (MUFAs) can lower LDL cholesterol without affecting HDL cholesterol nor do they raise triglycerides.

Monounsaturated fats possess antioxidant properties that can neutralize free radicals that is formed when LDLs are oxidized.

MUFAs are primarily found in fruits such as avocados, and vegetables sources including plant oils like canola and olive oil, and nuts such as walnuts, almonds, and pistachios and hazelnuts. Choose cold press oils over refined oils or processed cooking oil.

Monounsaturated fats are less prone to oxidation than polyunsaturated fats when heated.

Keep monounsaturated fats at a level of 10 to 15 percent of total calories.

Polyunsaturated Fats (Unrefined)

Polyunsaturated fats from unrefined or unprocessed oils help lower LDL but they also lower your HDL. Polyunsaturated fats can also be broken down into two types:

- Omega-6 polyunsaturated fats – these fats provide an essential fatty acid that our bodies need, but can't make. Vegetable oils like soy, sunflower, safflower are rich sources of polyunsaturated fats.

  They tend to be liquid at room temperature but can be made solid by hydrogenation to extend the shelf life of a product. This process changes the chemistry of the polyunsaturated fat into trans fatty acids, the fat to be avoided.

- Omega-3 polyunsaturated fats – these fats can be sourced from plants and cold water fish. Fish is a richer source of omega-3 fatty acids.

  Keep polyunsaturated fats at 5 to 10 percent of total calories.

Summary of Omega-3 and -6 Fat Sources

Monounsaturated Fat Sources	Omega-6 Polyunsaturated Fat Sources	Omega-3 Polyunsaturated Fat Sources

Nuts
Vegetable oils
Canola oil
Olive oil
High oleic
  safflower oil
Sunflower oil
Avocado
	Soybean oil
	Corn oil
	Safflower oil
		Soybean oil
		Canola oil
		Walnuts
		Flaxseed
		Fish: trout, herring
		  and salmon

INCREASE SOLUBLE FIBER IN YOUR DIET

Dietary fiber comes from the cell walls of plants, such as grains, nuts, beans, vegetables and fruits, and includes cellulose, lignin, pectins and gums.

Beta-Glucan

Research has shown that it is the beta-glucan in soluble fiber of cereals that plays an important role in helping lower Total cholesterol and LDL cholesterol. Beta-glucan is found in the cell walls of grains particularly from oats and barley and to a much lesser degree in rye and wheat. In general, experts recommend whole grains over processed or refined cereals.

This is how it works: Unlike starches, sugars and proteins, beta-glucan is not digested by the enzymes in the intestine. Instead, it transforms into a water soluble, non-digestible gel that coats the intestine. Here the sticky gel of the beta-glucan targets the LDL faction and dietary fat and removes them from the body. However, strangely it leaves the HDL alone.

Sources of Beta-Glucan

Oats

Beta-glucan is the component of soluble fiber common in oats that can be separated from the oat grain by selective milling.

Based on more than 50 human clinical studies, the United States Food and Drug Administration have allowed manufacturers to claim that the soluble fiber in the form of beta-glucan in oat bran, oat flour or rolled oats, could lower LDL but not the HDL cholesterol.

Adding beta-glucan to the diet has been shown to reduce blood cholesterol levels by up to 10 percent. However, if you stop your daily intake of beta-glucan, your blood cholesterol will return to the level where you began.

Barley

A new study indicates that barley beta-glucan has cholesterol-lowering properties similar to those of oats (*American Journal of Clinical Nutrition,* 2004; 80: 1185–93).

In barley, the beta-glucans are found throughout the entire kernel, whereas in most other grains, they're concentrated in the outer bran layer and can thus easily be lost in processing.

Soluble barley fiber from barley flakes, barley flour, and pearl barley are rich in beta-glucan. Pearl barley is sold in most supermarkets. Barley flour, flakes and grits may be found in health food stores.

Barley is a commonly used commercial ingredient in prepared foods such as breakfast cereals, soups, breads, cookies, crackers and snack bars.

Aim to eat at least 6 gm of beta-glucan daily for best results. The other rich sources of soluble fibers are dried beans and peas, flax seed, fruits such as oranges and apples, vegetables such as carrots, and whole grains such as wild rice, brown rice, whole wheat and whole rye.

Psyllium Seed Husks
It is a potent natural soluble fiber from the husk of the psyllium seed of the Plantago ovata plant. The seeds are covered by husks, which is the part of the plant used in foods.

The psyllium husk is another good source of water soluble fiber, similar to fiber found in grains such as oats and barley. But the amount of soluble fiber in psyllium is much higher than oat bran.

In 1998, the U.S. Food and Drug Administration gave the green light for psyllium husks to be used in food and dietary supplements to help people to maintain healthy cholesterol and blood lipid profile.

A diet low in saturated fats and cholesterol plus psyllium, can reduce Total cholesterol levels by 4 percent and LDL cholesterol by 7 percent. It works by reducing absorption of blood cholesterol and bile acids from the intestine into the blood stream and this action helps lower blood cholesterol levels.

Standard preparations of psyllium are available in dry seed or husk form, to be mixed with water as needed. But you may also find them in capsules and powder form.

If you are on any form of medication, it is recommended that you take it one hour before or two hours after taking psyllium. This is because psyllium can reduce the absorption and effectiveness of the medication you are taking.

INCLUDE PLANT STEROLS AND STANOLS

Plant sterols and stanols are the plant kingdom's equivalent of cholesterol. They act as a structural component of plant cell membrane just as cholesterol is an important component of the human cell membrane.

Research shows that plant sterols and stanols can lower cholesterol.

Sterols and stanols can be found in natural plants or they can, through a chemical process, enable manufacturers to incorporate them into a variety of our foods.

Sterols
Sterols are unsaturated components of vegetable oils and fats. It has a structure that is very similar to that of

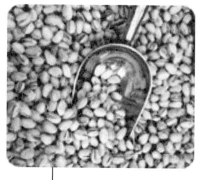

cholesterol.

Sterols of plants are called *phytosterols*. There are over 60 types of plant sterol, but the most common form is beta-sitosterol.

Sterols of plants are cholesterol-like substances that are naturally present in small quantities in a variety of fruits, vegetables, nuts, seeds, cereals, legumes, vegetable oils, and other plant sources.

Stanols

Stanols, unlike sterols, are saturated components of vegetable oils and fats. Like the sterols, stanols have a structure that is very similar to that of cholesterol.

Stanols (phytostanols) are present in trace levels in similar plant foods found in sterols.

Foods Fortified with Plant Sterols or Stanols

Since plant sterols and stanols have powerful cholesterol-lowering properties, and they occur naturally in small amounts, many manufacturers have started to incorporate concentrated levels into a variety of foods such as margarine spread, cereals, snack foods, cocoa-flavored bars, salad dressing, milk, yogurt and mayonnaise, some cooking oils, and concentrated juices.

You will find an array of foods fortified with sterols and stanols in your regular grocery store shelves. Regular and light margarines are available, both with only trace amounts of trans fatty acids.

Learn to read labels if you want to find out whether the food you are buying is enriched with plant sterols or stanols. Plant sterol enriched products will carry the words "plant sterols", "plant sterol esters" or "phytosterol esters". The label should include the total amount of plant sterols added in grams per serving of food.

A significant body of research has shown that plant sterols are safe even when consumed in amounts well above 3 grams per day. However, there is no increase in the cholesterol lowering effect of plant sterols when eaten in amounts above approximately 3 grams per day, say researchers.

If you use butter or margarine now, just switch over to one of these sterol-fortified spreads if your cholesterol numbers are at unhealthy levels.

Commercial Brands
Here are some better known commercial brands fortified with sterols and stanols:

Benecol: Margarine spread, salad dressing and yogurt. The cholesterol lowering ingredient is from plant stanols, derived from the wood pulp of pine trees.

Take Control: A margarine spread. The chief ingredient is from plant sterols derived from soybeans.

Phytrol: A margarine spread. Major ingredient is

plant sterols extracted from wood pulp.

Fortified sterol and stanol products are *not* calorie free and more is not necessarily better! It is best to consume them as part of a healthy, low-fat diet and in the amounts recommended by manufacturers.

How Do Sterols and Stanols Work in the Body?
The sterols/stanols work by blocking the absorption of cholesterol in the small intestine and also by blocking the re-absorption of cholesterol manufactured in the liver. The result: Cholesterol is excreted from the body, and this reduces our Total and LDL cholesterol levels in the body.

Clinical studies show they can lower LDL by 6 to 15 percent, without lowering HDL or triglycerides. Plant stanols/sterols do not interfere with cholesterol lowering medications.

The National Cholesterol Education Program recommends that people who have high cholesterol get 2 grams of stanols a day from margarine enriched with stanols but not as a replacement for diet, lifestyle change or prescribed lipid-lowering medications.

Limitations of Sterols/Stanols
Because plant sterols lower cholesterol absorption, they can also lower the absorption of some fat-soluble vitamins, in particular, levels of beta-carotene and vitamin E.

Plant sterols will only actively prevent the absorption of cholesterol if consumed on a regular basis, preferably at least two meals a day.

Research aside, some experts say people are better off getting their nutrients from whole foods. Whole foods offer a complex combination of nutrients that work together in ways we don't fully understand.

Patients on cholesterol-lowering medication should use these foods in consultation with their health care provider. Children or pregnant and breast-feeding women should avoid taking sterols or stanols.

What Health Authorities Say
The National Cholesterol Education Program recommends that people with high cholesterol could eat foods fortified with 2 grams of plant sterols or stanols a day. This chemical structure allows sterols to compete with, and slow down, cholesterol absorption in the intestines.

Most sterols-fortified foods contain at least 1 gram of plant sterols per serving. Please read the portion size and usage direction on the labels for details. It is important to note that plant sterols are not for everyone.

The U.S. Food and Drug Administration has also endorsed these products "as part of a dietary strategy to reduce the risk of coronary heart disease."

The American Heart Association doesn't recommend sterol and stanol-fortified foods for everyone. Instead, it suggests that only people who need to lower their cholesterol (over 4.1) or who had a heart attack should use them.

One important study published in the *New England Journal of Medicine* of people with high cholesterol found that less than an ounce of stanol-fortified margarine a day could lower "bad" LDL cholesterol by 14 percent.

"Eating sterol and stanol-containing foods is an easy way to lower your LDL cholesterol, which helps reduce the risk of heart disease," says Ruth Frechman, RD, a spokeswoman for the American Dietetic Association (ADA).

Make sure the margarines fortified with sterols/stenols contain only traces of trans fatty acids.

AVOID FOODS RICH IN CHOLESTEROL

The only foods that contain cholesterol directly and can raise your blood cholesterol numbers are those derived from animals including meats, poultry, fish, egg yolks, cheese, butter, liver and other organ meats, full-fat dairy products, high-fat processed meats, fried foods, steak, bacon, spareribs, sausages, hot dogs, hamburger, luncheon meats. The safe range of cholesterol intake is 200-400 milligrams per day. Here is a detailed list of foods containing cholesterol:

Food Sources	Cholesterol per 100 g of food in mg
Beef – loin, raw	70
Beef – on average, raw	59
Beef – ribs, raw	58
Beef – tongue, raw	108
Butter – ordinary	220
Bone marrow	3000
Camembert cheese – whole fat	73
Caviar	50
Cheddar cheese – whole fat	90
Chicken – breast, meat only, raw	64
Chicken – dark meat, meat only, raw	83
Chicken – liver, raw	380
Chicken eggs – whole, raw	600
Chicken eggs – yolk, raw	1790
Cod – smoked	50
Cod-liver oil	850
Cottage cheese – whole fat	37
Cream – 20% fat	66
Cream – 35% fat	120
Dried milk – powder, whole fat	109
Duck – on average, raw	76
Edam cheese – fat	71
Emmentaler cheese – fat	83
Goose – on average, raw	80
Hen – on average, raw	81
Herring – raw	64
Herring in oil	52
Herring in tomato sauce	50
Horse – on average, meat only, raw	75
Ice-cream	34
Kefir – natural, 2% fat	8
Lard	95

Mackerel – smoked	70
Meat paté	130
Milk – cow, 3,5% fat	14
Milk – goat	11
Milk – sheep	27
Mutton – leg, raw	78
Mutton – meat only, raw	78
Perch – raw	38
Pork – belly, raw	60
Pork – ham, raw	60
Pork – hearts, raw	140
Pork – kidney, raw	375
Pork – loin, raw	69
Pork – liver, raw	300
Pork – on average, raw	61
Pork – spare ribs, raw	66
Pork fat	99
Pork sausage	100
Rabbit – on average, raw	65
Salmon – raw	360
Sardines in oil	120
Shrimps – raw	152
Trout – raw	55
Tuna in oil	55
Turkey – breast, meat and skin, raw	65
Turkey – dark meat, meat and skin, raw	72
Turkey – on average	68
Veal – leg, raw	71
Veal – meat only, raw	71
Veal brain	2830
Yogurt – natural, 2% fat	8

DITCH THE UGLY TRANS FATS

Trans Fatty Acids

Over the last several decades, partially hydrogenated oils became a mainstay in margarines, commercially baked goods, and snack foods.

The use of partially hydrogenated vegetable oils was promoted as a healthy alternative to saturated fats when researched showed that it was "artery clogging." The last 15 years of nutrition research has shown that this "man-made fats" is worse than saturated fats for heart health.

Trans fatty acids (also called trans fats or hydrogenated fats) are solid fats produced by heating liquid vegetable oils in the presence of metal catalysts and hydrogen. Also, trans fats can be found in places that do not require labeling, like restaurants and cafeterias.

Trans fatty acids, as opposed to saturated fats, have been shown by researchers such as Enig, Mann and Fred Kummerow to be a major cause of atherosclerosis, coronary heart disease, cancer and other degenerative diseases.

What Do Researchers Say About Trans Fat?

"We are taking a risk when we consume food and products that contain trans fats; this is an invisible and dangerous ingredient that

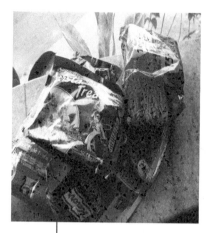

increases the risk of heart disease, stroke and high blood pressure – it had to be eliminated," says Tony Mendoza, California Assemblyman.

Trans fats lower HDL (good) cholesterol and increase LDL (bad) cholesterol. They increase rigidity and clogging of arteries, causes insulin resistance, and contributes to Type 2 diabetes and other health problems.

Trans fats also increase triglyceride levels in the blood, adding to your risk of cardiovascular disease.

"Trans fats should make up less than one percent of calories for Americans over two years old," according to the American Heart Association.

Why Manufacturers Love Trans Fats

This is an ideal fat for the food industry to work with because of its high melting point, its creamy and smooth texture, its reusability in deep-fat frying and it does not oxidize easily. Trans fats also extend the shelf life of a product. Trans fats make your crackers and popcorn buttery, French fries crispy, fish sticks crunchy, and pies and pastries that melt-in-your mouth.

Trans Fats in Food Labels

Packaged food products in the United States and Canada are now required to list the grammage of trans fatty acids contained within one serving of the product. A product claiming to have "zero" trans fats per serving does not necessarily mean it does not contain any trans fats. It can actually contain up to a half gram. If a product's list of ingredients contains the words "partially hydrogenated vegetable oil" or "vegetable shortening," the product contains trans fats.

Many margarines and spreads are now available with low or zero levels of trans fats, but they are less suitable for cooking and baking.

Since 2006, all manufacturers of food containing trans fatty acids have it on their nutrition labels. Labels that say "0 grams of Trans Fats" just simply mean the food still contains trans fats amounting to 0.5 g of trans fats.

Major Sources of Trans Fats for American Adults

Food Source of Trans Fatty Acids	Daily Intake Percentage
Cakes, cookies, crackers, pies, bread	40%
Butter, milk products, cheese, beef and lamb	21%
Margarine	17%
French fries and fried potatoes	8%
Potato chips, corn chips and popcorn	5%
Shortening (e.g., "Crisco")	4%
Salad dressings	3%

| Breakfast cereals | 1% |
| Candy | 1% |

Banning of Trans Fats

The State of California will be banning its restaurants from serving foods containing trans fats in 2010. By 2011, baked foods containing trans fats will also be disallowed.

Since July 2008, New York has banned trans fats in all its 24,000 restaurants, high-end eateries to fast-food joints. Philadelphia and Boston are following suit.

Wendy's, America's third-largest burger chain, was the first of the big fast-food chains to revamp her cooking oil blend to reduce trans fats in its chicken and French fries by an average of 95 percent, and even reduced saturated-fat content by an average of 20 percent. Food companies like Kraft and Starbucks have joined the bandwagon. KFC is also working to remove trans fats from its fried products.

The World Health Organization (WHO) has strongly recommended to the governments around the world to phase out the use of partially hydrogenated oils if trans fat labeling alone does not spur any significant reductions.

With the information we already know about the ugly side of trans fat, we should seriously consider to eliminate trans fats from our daily diet.

Here is what you can do to lower trans fat intake:

- Choose liquid vegetable oils, or choose a soft tub margarine that contains little or no trans fats.

- Avoid eating commercially prepared baked foods such as cookies, pies, donuts, snack foods, processed foods, and fast foods.

- When foods containing partially hydrogenated oils can't be avoided, choose products that list the partially hydrogenated oils near the end of the ingredient list.

- To avoid trans fats in restaurants, don't order deep-fried foods or desserts.

- Use liquid plant oils for cooking and baking. Olive, canola, and other plant-based oils are rich in heart-healthy unsaturated fats as long as they are not refined.

- Switch from butter to soft tub margarine. Choose a product that has zero grams of trans fats, and scan the ingredient list to make sure it does not contain partially hydrogenated oils.

Minimize Your Triglycerides Intake
It is important to keep tab of your triglycerides (fat) as they are associated with high LDL and low HDL. If you consume excess calories regardless from any source – carbohydrates, fats or protein, your body will

transform the excess calories into triglycerides for storage as body fat.

To lower triglycerides, try to:

- Eat a healthy diet low in saturated fats and trans fatty acids. Trim visible fats from meats.

- Use lower fat dairy or cheese instead of regular version.

- Include high-fiber foods such as whole grains, oatmeal and fruits.

- Reduce intake of refined carbohydrates like white sugar and white flour. Eat carbohydrates based on the Glycemic Index and Glycemic Load.

- Include omega-3-rich foods from cold water fish such as salmon, fish oils and flax seed. Fish oil can lower our triglycerides by as much as 65 percent, lower LDL cholesterol, and lower blood pressure.

- Do not over-eat; watch portion size when eating out.

- Use trans-fat-free margarine if you prefer margarine.

- One of the best fats you can add to your diet is

extra virgin olive oil. Extra virgin is the least processed olive oil, making it as close to natural as you can get. This amazing oil helps to decrease LDL and increase HDL levels.

TOP TEN FOODS THAT CAN LOWER EXCESS LDL IN THE BODY

Soy Foods: The basics include tofu, soy nuts, tempeh, soybeans, soy flour, and enriched soymilk. The isoflavones and soluble fiber, the health component in soybeans, act like human hormones that can lower LDL cholesterol and raise HDL cholesterol.

Beans: Particularly kidney, navy, pinto, black, chickpea, or butter beans. Beans and legumes are an excellent source of soluble fiber and high in vegetable protein. Properly combined beans become an excellent substitute for red meat protein that is high in saturated fat.

Cold Water Fish: It is a good source of protein and omega-3 fatty acids, which has been shown to lower LDL cholesterol and raise HDL cholesterol and lower triglyceride. To get the most omega-3s, choose salmon, white albacore tuna canned in water, rainbow trout, anchovies, herring, sardines, and mackerel.

Avocado: The American Heart Association recommends that you get up to 15 percent of your daily calories from heart healthy monounsaturated fats that can increase your levels of HDL cholesterol.

Avocados are rich in oleic acid, a monounsaturated fat known to help lower cholesterol. One recent study found that people with moderately high cholesterol levels who ate a diet high in avocados for one week had significant drops in Total and LDL cholesterol levels, and a 11 percent increase in the good HDL cholesterol.

Garlic: Garlic contains the chemical allicin which helps lower the blood clotting properties of blood and has received attention over recent years for its usefulness in lowering cholesterol levels.

Garlic is helpful in preventing and reversing heart and cardiovascular disease by lowering Total cholesterol, LDL and triglycerides while raising HDL. Chop up and toss on pizza, in soups, or on side dishes.

Cinnamon: A study published in the journal *Diabetes Care* found that half a teaspoon of cinnamon a day reduces triglycerides, LDL, Total cholesterol level and significantly reduces blood sugar levels in people with type 2 diabetes.

Nuts: Almonds, hazelnuts and walnuts are rich sources of monounsaturated fats, fiber, antioxidants and plant sterols that can significantly reduce blood cholesterol and also help keep blood vessels healthy and elastic. Nuts also have vitamin E, magnesium, copper, and phytochemicals.

Tea: A cup of green or black tea contains more antioxidants than a serving of any fruit or vegetable. Flavonoids, the major antioxidants in tea, help prevent the oxidation of LDL cholesterol that leads to plaque formation on artery walls.

Apples: It contains three important compounds to lower cholesterol:

Pectin: A soluble fiber that reduces the amount of LDL cholesterol made in the liver.

Insoluble fiber: Works to remove LDL from the body.

Quercetin: An antioxidant that helps LDL cholesterol from being oxidized by free radicals.

A recent study conducted in Finland concluded that eating three apples a day for three months can help you drop your cholesterol level by 20 points.

Grapes: A rich source of flavonoids such as quercetin and resveratrol. Grapes may protect against CVD by improving cholesterol levels and decreasing LDL oxidation as well as exerting beneficial effects on blood clotting.

Whole Grains and Oats: A five-year Insulin Resistance Athersclerosis Study showed that people whose diets contain the most whole grains "had the thinnest carotid artery walls and showed the slowest progression in artery wall thickness."

Five to ten grams of soluble fiber in oatmeal can help reduce LDL by about five percent. Eating 1.5

cups of cooked oatmeal provides 4.5 grams of fiber, that is enough to lower your cholesterol.

When eating foods containing oats, however, be sure to always eat whole grain oats.

The list suggested is not exhaustive as there are many other good foods that can help people with elevated cholesterol.

Overall Goal Guide

The US National Cholesterol and Education Program (May 2001) suggests that adults use diet to lower their cholesterol levels before trying medication. The report encourages the consumption of foods rich in soluble fibers such as cereal grains, beans, peas, legumes and a variety of fruits and vegetables to help lower cholesterol levels.

Ideally aim for a diet containing about 25 percent calories from fat, divided as follows: Polyunsaturated fat (10 percent), monounsaturated fat (10 percent), saturated/trans fat (no more than 5 percent).

What to Do When Eating Out

If you're eating healthy food at home to keep cholesterol in check, don't blow it when you eat out. Restaurant food can be loaded with saturated fat, calories, and sodium. Even healthy choices may come in super-size portions. Try these tips to stay on track:

- Choose broiled, baked, steamed, and grilled foods – not fried

- Get sauces on the side
- Practice portion control

Action Diary

Since our main goal is to reduce saturated fat and limit other fats too, a diet diary is needed. Most of us have no idea how much fat is in the different foods that we eat. I want you to do two things. Buy a book that lists the calories and grams of saturated fat in various foods. Your goal is to keep the saturated fat intake down to below seven percent of your needed calories a day.

The second thing I want you to do is buy a notebook of some sort in which to keep your diary. Write down everything that goes into your mouth, especially your intake of calories and saturated fat. The dairy is to keep us honest and to make us very aware of which foods contain the greatest amounts of fat. I call my diary "D.I.E.T." The letters stand for "Did I Eat That?" It keeps me honest!

If you keep up with your food intake and fat grams for four weeks, you will automatically become very discriminating in your food choices. Look at your saturated fat and calories as money in the bank. As you eat each meal, you make withdrawals from your daily fat/calorie account. You only have an allowance of so much to spend, so budget and spend wisely. One person actually kept her diary in a check registry! It was quite effective.

A parting advice on diet – when eating, choose food for health, NOT FOR TASTE.

Key #3

Increase Your
High-Density Lipoprotein

Reducing your Total cholesterol will definitely lower your heart attack risk. But, raising your HDL will dramatically lower your risk! Besides, exercise lowers your triglycerides level, and may also lower your LDL cholesterol level.

Here are some ways you can take to increase your HDL cholesterol:

EXERCISE YOUR WAY TO HEALTH

Remember, it is never too old or too late to start exercising.

If you are over 40, it is advisable that you go through a medical examination and a treadmill stress test before you embark on any vigorous exercise.

If you have been sedentary for a while, begin any exercise at a slow pace and gradually increase the intensity. To benefit from any form of exercise, it must be done regularly.

Research has shown that exercise can generally help improve your cholesterol although the benefits will vary among individuals.

Below are some established facts based on research but I will not bore you with the details:

- A few months of regular brisk walking can increase your HDL cholesterol.

- Even moderate exercise like walking and slow jogging for 30 minutes three times a week can help increase your HDL.

- Survivors of a heart attack who participate in a moderate exercise program not only increase their HDL but lower their risk of another heart attack in the future.

- There is a limit to which exercise can help increase your HDL level. Research has shown that some people's HDL may remain steady whilst others decline.

- People who are not physically active may lower their HDL significantly.

- Smoking can have a negative impact on HDL.

- Anaerobic exercise such as weight-lifting or sprinting does not increase HDL.

- Exercise benefits people of all ages. Older people will enjoy the same increase in HDL as younger people.

However, exercise combined with a low fat and low cholesterol diet is the best starting point for a program to control cholesterol successfully than diet or exercise alone.

Aerobic Exercise

Each time you exercise, always spend a minimum of three to five minutes to warm up. After you have completed the aerobic phase, it must be followed by a cool-down period. Keep moving around for about five minutes after completing your exercise.

Consistency, intensity and duration of an aerobic exercise can lead to a leaner body weight. This has a tremendous impact on your HDL and Total cholesterol.

Aerobic exercise can have a direct impact on not only your HDL but also your Total cholesterol/ HDL ratio. However, its impact on Total cholesterol is inconsistent.

Here are some aerobic exercises you can incorporate into your exercise program in order to help you increase your HDL.

Walking

Number one, by far, is walking. Don't panic! You can count adequate "strolling" among this. Let's do strolling first because it sounds less intimidating.

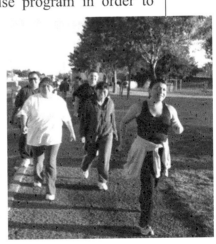

Researchers at the

Cooper Institute for Aerobics Research in Dallas, Texas, concluded that you can raise HDL without vigorous exercise. This study was accepted for publication in the *Journal of the American Medical Association.*

The participants involved 59 healthy women divided into four groups as follows:

- GROUP ONE: Walked fast (five miles per hour, almost a run)
- GROUP TWO: Walked briskly (four miles an hour)
- GROUP THREE: Walked moderately (three miles an hour)
- GROUP FOUR: Remained sedentary

Each walking group covered three miles, five days a week for six months. Results: The first two groups were just about equal in HDL gains, and their aerobic capacities were close. Even the slow walkers got some gain. So, you have a choice: Go fast for a shorter period of time or slower for a longer period of time.

Is this really "new" information? No. "Walking is man's best medicine," said Hippocrates in 400 BC! It worked then and it will work for you now. Equipment needed: Comfortable shoes and a determination to do it!

Raising your HDL is extremely powerful. Several good studies have indicated that you reduce your heart attack risk by an awesome seven percent for each point you elevate your HDLs above 50.

For older people or those who need to walk more slowly, slower walking (two miles per hour) can also offer many advantages.

Running

If you really want to "run up" the good cholesterol, it takes a little more effort. A team led by George Town University researcher Peter Kokkinos, Ph.D., measured cholesterol levels in some 2,900 men aged 30 to 64. Most were runners; the rest were healthy but sedentary. When the researchers charted the running mileage and HDL levels, they found that for every additional mile they ran, HDL rose by about 0.008. Those who covered the most distance had the highest HDL. The intermediate group had HDL levels 11 percent higher than the non-runners.

"Women who run more than 10 miles a week have slimmer waists, narrower hips, lower blood pressure, and higher levels of 'good' HDL cholesterol than do those who exercise less intensely," says Paul Williams, PhD, a researcher at the University of California, Berkeley, and lead investigator of the landmark National Runners' Health Study of more than 9,000 people.

Based on the study, researchers recommended the equivalent of running 7 to 14 miles a week at a moderate pace. That's about 30 minutes of exercise three to five times a week.

For cardiovascular conditioning it is preferable to run long and slow instead of short and fast.

To avoid injuries follow some of the tips recommended for jogging.

Jogging

Jogging is running at brisk, trotting pace that has a high impact on particularly your heels and knee joints.

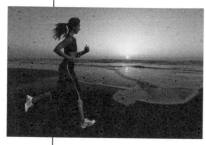

Jogging burns more calories per mile than walking. Jogging helps burn calories from the hip, thighs and abdominal area and helps improve your HDL and lower your LDL, thus improving your cardiovascular health.

Before you start, consult your physician, especially when you have been sedentary. Your physician is the best person to evaluate your physical condition.

But jogging is not without risks, especially if you have a heart condition. During a vigorous session, the heart can develop an irregular beat, blood pressure can rise to a dangerous level or plaque from a partly clogged artery can break off and stop blood flow.

What gears do you need for jogging? The first priority is a pair of jogging shoes that can absorb impact shocks. The shoes must provide all round protection and have good cushioning soles especially to the ankles. Buy your jogging shoes from a reputable source.

A garden or a joggers' track is the best place to start jogging. It is best to avoid running on busy roads.

The best time is early in the morning.

Here are some helpful tips to avoid injury especially to your knee joints as jogging is a high impact sport:

- Do some stretching and swing your arms before you begin your jog.

- Land on the heel for balance and as you proceed, push from the toes.

- Swing your arms in matching strides to your jogging trots.

- Don't clench your fists.

- Don't hunch when you jog, instead holding chest thrust forward. It keeps lungs expanded.

- Increase speed and distance gradually.

- Carry cold water with you to quench thirst while jogging.

- Always end with 5-10 minutes of totally relaxed posture. Relax by taking deep and slow breaths. This helps upward blood circulation.

Swimming
The health benefits of swimming are almost

unmatched by any other sport.

Regular swimming works your whole body, builds endurance, muscle strength, posture, flexibility and cardio-vascular fitness as swimming improves your body's use of oxygen without overworking your heart.

- It increases the HDL in your blood, protecting you against heart attack.

- Swimming does burn calories at a rate of about 3 calories a mile per pound of body weight.

- The greatest advantage about swimming over many other sports is that it's a low impact exercise. The risk for swimming injuries is minimal as there's no stress on your bones, joints or connective tissues without jarring or tearing it.

- Improves blood pressure. Studies have shown that swimming can help reduce and possibly prevent high blood pressure which lowers your risk for heart disease and stroke.

- Great way to relieve stress. Swimming is relaxing as it allows more oxygen to flow to your muscles.

Cycling
According to the British Heart Foundation, cycling at

least 20 miles per week reduces the risk of coronary heart disease to less than half that for non-cyclists.

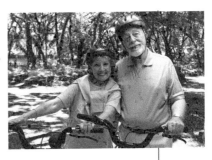

Research shows that cycling can lower LDL levels and significantly increase HDL. Cycling reduces the risk of serious conditions such as heart disease, high blood pressure, obesity and the most common form of diabetes.

Cycling improves blood circulation by carrying oxygen-rich blood to all the muscles of the body. The heavy breathing experienced in cycling increases the intake of oxygen, making it an effective aerobic exercise.

The health benefits of cycling far outweigh the physical risk associated with cycling such as an accident. It is a fantastic workout that not only enables you to derive pleasure, but it can help you shed off those extra calories and get rid of flabby abs.

On the other hand, if you don't like cycling outdoor you can resort to a stationary cycle found in most gyms or you can purchase one.

Racquet Games
Tennis really provides cardiovascular benefits and is a great physical activity. You are working all of your muscle groups, getting your heart rate up plus you're toning as well.

The game of tennis helps you exercise your

muscles, burn calories and help lower blood pressure
— all of which adds up to a significantly reduced risk
of heart attack or stroke.

GET YOUR WEIGHT DOWN

A recent guideline on May 15, 2001 by the National
Cholesterol Education Program (NCEP) confirms
beyond doubt the need for weight control, physical
activity and intensified use of nutrition to lower risk of
heart disease. Weight control and greater physical
activity improves your HDL.

Being overweight tends to lead to unhealthy
cholesterol levels. Losing weight can lower your bad
LDL cholesterol and triglycerides. It also can raise
your good HDL cholesterol.

Body Mass Index

Your body mass index (BMI) is a good indicator as to
whether you are in an unhealthy weight range. To
calculate your BMI just divide your weight by your
height squared.

A healthy BMI is 20-25. At 25-30 means you
are overweight and above 30 indicates obesity. Greater
than 40 is extreme obesity.

Waist Circumference

The BMI focuses on weight rather than where the fat
is distributed in the body. Experts are now
recommending measuring waist circumference or

waist-to-hip ratio as an additional tool to measure obesity.

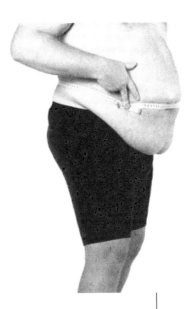

Your waist circumference is also a good indicator of how much fat is in your abdomen. The bigger your waist circumference, the more intra-abdominal fats you have.

Research shows that there is a higher incidence of coronary heart disease and diabetes in people who are "apple-shaped", or who store weight around their abdomens, than in those who are more "pear-shaped", with fat mostly around the hip and thighs.

If you are a man, you are obese if your waist circumference is more than 35.5 inches and, in the case of woman, a waist circumference exceeding 31.5 inches

Waist-to-Hip Ratio

By World Health Standard, you are obese if your waist-to-hip ratio is over 1 for men and over 0.8 for women.

Simply divide the size of the waist by the size of the hip to get this ratio.

INCREASE YOUR CONSUMPTION OF COLD WATER FISH

Mackerel, haddock, anchovies, sardines, tuna and some salmon, all contain an unusual fatty acid called eicosapentaenoic acid or EPA for short. The EPA actually lowers triglycerides. As you recall, high HDL is associated with low triglycerides. This is the reason fish is in your food choices. It's hard to consume as much of these blue skinned fish as you need.

The human body can make most of the types of fats it needs from other fats or raw materials but the essential omega-3 fatty acids, you must get them from your food.

What makes omega-3 fats special? They are an integral part of cell membranes throughout the body. They provide the starting point for making hormones that regulate blood clotting, contraction and relaxation of artery walls, and inflammation.

The strongest evidence for a beneficial effect of omega-3 fats has to do with heart disease. These fats appear to help the heart beat at a steady pace and not veer into a dangerous or potentially fatal erratic rhythm. Such arrhythmias cause most of the 500,000-plus cardiac deaths that occur each year in the United States.

Omega-3 fats also lower blood pressure and heart rate, improve blood vessel function, and, at higher doses, lower triglycerides and may ease inflammation, which plays a role in the development of atherosclerosis.

Sources of Omega-3 Fatty Acids

You can get your supply of omega-3 fatty acids from polyunsaturated fats from two sources:

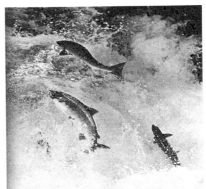

- Eicosapentaenoic acid (EPA) and docosahexaenoic acid (DHA) come mainly from fish, especially salmon, and are sometimes called marine omega-3s.

- Alpha-linolenic acid (ALA) is also found in vegetable oils and nuts (especially walnuts), leafy vegetables, and some animal fat, especially in grass-fed animals. The human body generally uses ALA for energy, and conversion into EPA and DHA is very limited.

INCREASE YOUR CONSUMPTION OF SOLUBLE FIBER

Soluble fiber seems to actually target LDL cholesterol and leave the HDL alone. So, as you lower the Total cholesterol in this way, your ratio improves because the HDL stays high or even goes up a point or two. For more information on soluble fiber see Key #2 on using diet to control your cholesterol.

EAT MORE OFTEN
TO LOWER CHOLESTEROL

"If you are already eating well and want to have further benefit, at least for cholesterol, dividing what you eat into more frequent meals may have additional benefits. The more frequently the better – four, five or six (meals) spread out over the day, so smaller amounts are eaten more frequently," says Dr Kay-Tee Khaw of the University of Cambridge. This research is published in the *British Medical Journal*.

A recent guideline on May 15, 2001 by the National Cholesterol Education Program (NCEP) confirms beyond doubt the need for weight control, physical activity and intensified use of nutrition to lower risk of heart disease. Weight control and greater physical activity improves your HDL and, for some, LDL.

DO NOT SMOKE ANYTHING!

This is good advice for anyone. Numerous experts have been asked, "What is the one thing I can do to increase my healthy life span?" The answer is consistent: "Do not smoke." Even second hand smoke may lower HDL.

"Without question, cigarette increases your risk of heart disease and upsets your cholesterol levels," says Dr Kenneth Cooper of The Aerobic

Centre in Dallas.

The famous Framingham Heart Study as far back as 1970 has reported that smoking lowers blood level of HDL. Recent research has shown that:

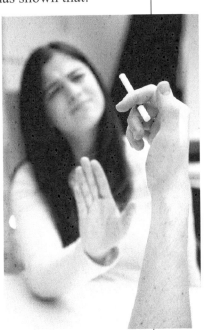

- Smoking conclusively lowers HDL.

- Smokers are more prone to developing atherosclerosis than non-smokers.

- The more cigarettes a person smokes, the more HDL will decline.

- The decline in HDL is greater in female than male smokers.

DON'T DRINK ALCOHOL

Some research has shown that drinking alcohol in limited amount is good for the heart. Some claim drinking beer or liquor can cut chances of a heart attack by half and others claim drinkers have stronger hearts.

Most researchers tend to believe that the

dangers of alcohol outweigh the benefits. Because of the dangers liquor place on our health, I believe you should take other safer routes to raise your HDL like diet and exercise which we have discussed at length.

MANAGE YOUR DAILY STRESS LEVEL

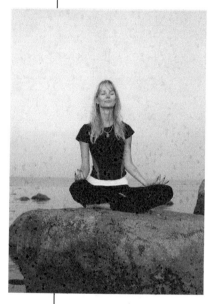

We need stress to survive but it is chronic stress that can endanger our health. But coping with stress by smoking, eating unhealthy foods and remaining sedentary is not the right way to manage your stress level.

Learning to relax and control your stress will not only help you to enjoy life more, but it will be better for your heart health in the long run.

There are many ways to get your stress levels down. Below are some ways that can help you to relax and reduce your stress levels:

- List the things that trigger your stress. Pinning down the cause of your stress trigger is a big step forward. Try to relax in these situations.

- Build a social support network of friends and

family. Remember the wise saying: A trouble shared is a trouble halved.

- Learn stress coping strategies such as relaxation techniques, breathing exercises, meditation, yoga or massage.

- Take time out to unwind, even if it's just for five minutes. Try to do something else you enjoy. Don't work continuously for long hours and make sure you take a break from time to time to relax your mind.

- Taking regular exercise, such as gentle cycling, brisk walking or swimming or racquet games.

- Stop trying to do more than one thing at a time. Rank your work according to importance and try to plan ahead, instead of doing everything at the last minute. Prioritize your day and your work.

- Seek professional help during time of chronic stress.

- Don't be a perfectionist.

- Accept what you cannot change.

- Don't bottle up your anger or allow resentment

to fester.
- Learn to say no sometimes.

- Learn to control your emotions before your emotions control you.

- Don't keep up with the Joneses – instead count your blessing.

- Be cheerful as it is a wonderful antidote for stress.

- Procrastination and stress are traveling companions.

- Be patient with yourself.

- Do not build up obstacles in your imagination.

- Be forgiving.

- Develop patience and gentleness into your character.

Key #4

Include
Cholesterol-Lowering
Supplements

F ood supplements are no longer an option in our diets. There are certain nutrients critical to protect us from heart disease and other dreaded killers, such as some forms of cancer. We cannot conveniently get several of these nutrients from our diets in the amounts needed for protection. One nutrient, vitamin E, is impossible to obtain in adequate amounts. Supplements are essential!

Dietary supplements often compliment pharmaceutical medications, and in some cases, the pharmaceutical drugs can cause a deficiency in a nutrient or substance important to human health.

SOLUBLE FIBER SUPPLEMENT

If you find difficulty in following a high fiber diet as discussed earlier, you may need to add a fiber supplement to your diet as it is a key player in our heart disease prevention program.

This may amaze you: A soluble fiber supplement will reduce cholesterol for most people even if they do nothing else. Why do I recommend a supplement? This is because even those who eat a very well-balanced diet, do not get enough of the key soluble fibers in their day-to-day diets.

I have read an excellent study concerning a supplement with four fibers. The study was headed by Dr William Haskell of Stanford University School of Medicine. The results of the study were reported in the American Journal of Cardiology. The researchers used a combination of pectin, psyllium, husks, guar, and locust bean gums.

In one part of the study, the soluble supplement was combined with weight loss and exercise, just as we recommended. The results were phenomenal. In just four weeks, the Total cholesterol of the participants was reduced by an average of 15 percent and LDL cholesterol was reduced by 22 percent!

Remember, for each one percent drop in Total cholesterol, you reduce your heart attack risk by two percent. The results of this study represent an amazing decrease in heart attack risk of 30 percent! Is this a lot? Yes! These results are even better than some of the LDL cholesterol-lowering drugs on the market, and without the side effects!

How Does This Work?
Cholesterol once made, cannot be broken down. It can only be removed from our body in the form of bile acids and cholesterol molecules.

Soluble fiber can bind bile acids (they contain

up to 95 percent cholesterol) in the small intestine to prevent them from being reabsorbed! It holds them and takes them to elimination. Not only that, but these fibers zero in on LDL and leave the good HDL alone.

The best time to take the supplement is just before your largest meal of the day. This meal will stimulate the most bile acid release from your gall bladder. You take the supplement first because you want these little cholesterol-binding sponges to be ahead of the food, ready to trap the cholesterol-rich bile. I would also take the supplement just before one other meal of the day. Studies indicate you need to take it at least twice a day for best results. If your cholesterol is really resistant, go to three servings a day for awhile.

There are two cautions to observe when you add fiber, be it from your diet or through supplements. First, add it slowly so your body can adjust to the additional fiber. If added too rapidly, it can produce gas. Also, be sure you get 8 to 10 glasses of purified water a day. Water helps fiber do its various jobs better.

MULTI-VITAMIN MINERAL

The first supplement to add to your daily food regime should be a multi-vitamin/mineral preparation. Personally, I feel everyone should be taking a multi. Numerous studies show that we do not get all the nutrients we need in necessary amounts.

No recognized vitamin or mineral in the Daily Value (DV) has been shown to have an adverse effect on your blood lipids, even if consumed slightly above the recommended levels. On the other hand, a shortage of some of these has been shown to put some of the lipid factors out of balance. A good general multi can be a good insurance for those nutrients that may be missing from your day-to-day diet.

OMEGA-3 FATTY ACID FROM FISH OIL

Eating fish oil seems to be the most realistic way of getting fish oil from the diet but unfortunately much of the fish we eat to-day are contaminated with organic mercury, PCBs and DDT. The solution to this dilemma is the use of fish oil in supplement form in which the above mentioned toxins have been removed.

We have known for years that native Eskimos who consume large quantities of blue-skinned, cold-water fish have a very low incidence of coronary heart disease. At first, this was just dismissed as genetics peculiar to this group. Then, some of these native Eskimos began consuming the American diet. Interestingly enough, they began to develop the same heart attack problems as we have.

We owe a lot of credit to a Danish epidemiologist by the name of Jorn Dyerberg. He made a careful study of the heart attack occurrences among Danes (who eat a diet like ours) and Greenland

Eskimos (who eat a diet high in EPA).

Heart disease is the number one killer of both Danes and North Americans. However, note the differences between these population groups and the Eskimos. The heart attack rate among North Americans is around 46 percent. But, the heart attack rate among Greenland Eskimos is less than eight percent ... a startling 38 percent difference! How does EPA do this?

Benefits

EPA "thins out" the blood. Through this process, there are fewer tendencies for the blood to develop clots, which can clog the vessels and cause a heart attack. Remember, in 90+ percent of heart attacks, a blood clot is the cause.

For most people, it will lower triglycerides, if high. High triglycerides are associated with low HDL (the good kind). If you can get your triglycerides down, it often results in the HDL moving up into a more healthy range.

It has, in some cases, even had a positive effect on high blood pressure. The mechanism of this is not understood. It could result from a slight widening of the blood vessels, or it could be due to the fact that EPA makes the blood more "slippery," causing it to flow more smoothly.

As a blood clot begins to form, one of the early stages is a clumping of the little cells that initiate the clot and the formation of tiny threads called fibrin. These pre-clots can cause blockage in blood vessels.

EPA actually helps to dissolve these clots (fibrinolysis) before they develop into a true, life-threatening clot.

The Ratio of Omega-6 to Omega-3

American diets are overloaded with omega-6 fatty acid and deficient in omega-3 fatty acid. The problem is the ratio of omega-6 to omega-3. The ratio in the current American diet is as high as 15:1. A healthier ratio would be 4:1 or better still 2:1.

Too much omega-6 fatty acid in your body will crowd out the benefits of omega-3 fatty acid. Without going into the complex subject of fat metabolism, you will not receive many of the wonderful benefits of omega-3 fats such as reduced risk of heart disease, cancer, stroke, Alzheimer's, arthritis and many other degenerative illnesses.

One caution: If you are taking a blood thinning drug, consult with your physician before taking EPA. The supplement could interfere with the drug.

GARLIC

In the past, the cry from the scientific community has been, "There's not enough evidence. Show us that garlic can stand up to scientific testing." Today, a growing number of researchers are taking up this challenge. Here are few of the results.

In a large study of 220 patients, the garlic group took 800 mg of powdered garlic for four months. The group experienced a 12 percent drop in cholesterol and a 17 percent drop in triglycerides. The placebo group had little change.

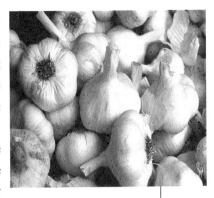

In Germany, where garlic is a licensed medicine for atherosclerosis, a study came out of Munich University. Patients were put on a low-fat diet, and the cholesterol fell 10 percent and stabilized. Garlic was added, and the cholesterol fell another 10 percent.

In a survey of dozens of studies, the results were remarkably consistent. With garlic, you can expect a drop in cholesterol of anywhere from 10 to 20 percent. It doesn't take much to do the job. In one study, 261 people were given 800 mg of dried garlic for 16 weeks. That is about the equivalent of a small clove of fresh garlic. There was an average drop of 10 percent in cholesterol.

A SOY PROTEIN SUPPLEMENT

You may have heard that North Americans consume too much protein. That information came from studies in the late 1970s and early 1980s, before we were told to take the vital health step of cutting down on fat, especially saturated fats. The problem is that most of our usual protein sources (meat, milk, cheese) have a lot of fats attached to them. As you lower the fats, you automatically lower the protein.

Susan Potter, Ph.D., at the University of Illinois at Urbana-Champaign, studied soy protein and heart disease. In testing various soy products and combinations, she found that isolated soy protein worked the best, resulting in a 12 percent drop in Total cholesterol and an 11.5 percent drop in LDL.

The researchers concluded: "The fact that a significant reduction is obtained by consuming only 50 grams a day of soy protein, sets a practical and achievable goal that would be beneficial in the treatment of high blood cholesterol and coronary artery disease."

In follow-up studies by Dr Potter's group, it was shown that even 25 grams (roughly one-half cup) of soy protein daily could result in significant reduction of cholesterol levels in those with elevated levels.

To put all of this in a nutshell, a paper was recently published in the New England Journal of Medicine summarizing the findings of 38, well-controlled studies on soy protein and cholesterol. Overall, there was about a 9 percent reduction in Total cholesterol and nearly a 13 percent reduction in the bad LDL.

How Does Soy Protein Work?
The build-up of plaque in arteries is thought to be caused by something that creates damage or alteration to the cells lining the coronary arteries. Many

researchers now strongly believe this injury may involve oxidation of LDL caused by free radicals.

We know cholesterol, specifically LDL cholesterol, is the culprit. Here is how it all works. Certain cells in the body are garbage disposals units. They line blood vessels and when something that does not belong in the blood vessels floats by; they grab it and eat it. These cells are called macrophages. "Macro" means big and "phage" means eater.

The "big eaters" consume the oxidized LDL cholesterol quite well, but the problem is they can't digest it. These cells become packed with fat and are called "foam cells." They become so stuffed that they cause the artery to bulge out into the lumen, the passageway of the artery. This protrusion attracts other cell debris, and we have the beginning of a fibrous bulging plaque that can cut off the flow of blood. Antioxidants help prevent the initial step – oxidation of the LDL.

A team of researchers from Hirosaki University School of Medicine recently tested this theory on animals. They divided rabbits into two groups. Both received the same diet, but one group was given soy protein and the other Probucol, a prescribed drug known to be an antioxidant.

In both groups the oxidation rate fell rapidly. In fact, the soy worked even better than the drug, Probucol, in preventing LDL oxidation! The results of the study were published in the Annals of the New York Academy of Sciences. "Thus, because soy proteins decreased the production of oxidized and deformed LDL, they are very useful in preventing the development of atherosclerotic diseases," said the authors of the study.

Still another way soy may help prevent heart problems is its amino acid composition. Although it is equal to meat and eggs as a complete protein, it has a different amino acid profile. Soy protein is lower in two essential amino acids (lysine and methionine) than meat. Studies have shown that when lysine is added to a soy diet, LDL levels can rise. Therefore, the ratio of the amino acids in soy may help prevent the formation of plaque.

The mechanism of just exactly how soy works its magic with cholesterol will be the subject of many studies. However, the main point to make is that soy works and works quite well!

VITAMIN E IS A MUST!

I routinely take a vitamin E food supplement, and I am careful to never miss a day. The research is too compelling. Vitamin E is an extremely powerful antioxidant and works especially well with cholesterol. We have covered the mechanics of LDL, oxidants and the artery clogging process under soy protein, so let's take a look at the research on vitamin E.

Dr Daniel Steinberg of the University of California at San Diego led a most revealing experiment. The scientists mixed LDL with macrophages in a test tube. In spite of their efforts, they could not force the macrophages to take up the LDL very quickly. Then they oxidized the LDL. "The macrophages took up the LDL 3 to 10 times faster," said Steinberg. When they added vitamin E (a strong antioxidant) to the same mix, the LDL was protected from being taken up by the macrophages. What a great discovery! If LDL isn't engulfed by macrophages, it cannot clog your arteries. This study was reported in the Journal of the American Medical Association. It has since been confirmed by numerous reports.

An ongoing Harvard University study headed by Dr Meir J. Stampfer reported on 87,000 female nurses. Those who took a supplement of vitamin E each day had about one-third less risk of heart attack or death from coronary disease than those who did not take supplements.

The Harvard study even made a believer out of the researcher. Dr Stampfer of the Harvard School of Public Health in Boston began the 87,000 nurse study expecting to disprove the idea that vitamin E could reduce the risk. He says, "It just didn't seem plausible that a simple maneuver like taking vitamin E would have such a profound effect."

This next study is extremely interesting. Last year, researchers reported evidence that the level of antioxidants in the blood may have more influence on heart disease than do classic coronary risk factors. In a comparison of 16 European populations of men, they found that a low vitamin E level was more closely related to the development of heart disease than high blood cholesterol and high blood pressure!

THE BATTLE CONTINUES WITH VITAMIN C

Several studies have shown that in populations where vitamin C intake is low, heart disease deaths are high, and where vitamin C intake is high, heart disease deaths are low.

Dr Ishwarlal Jialal, has done some work on vitamin C. He recently reported on the power of vitamin C as an antioxidant in the Journal *Atherosclerosis*. Dr Jialal did a study very similar to the one Dr Steinberg did with vitamin E. The results were astounding. Vitamin C cut the macrophage absorption of LDL by 93 percent! Jialal noted that smoking, diabetes and stress deplete the body's vitamin C. "All three are risk factors for heart disease, lending credence to the theory that oxidation plays a crucial role in the development of atherosclerosis," he said.

How do all these fit together? How can vitamin E and vitamin C do the same thing? I think this may be the answer. Vitamin E is a fat-soluble vitamin and works on reducing oxidation in the fatty parts of the cells. Vitamin C is a water-soluble vitamin and works in the aqueous parts of the cell. Both have a similar effect, but they just work in different cellular areas. If this is true, it would mean they have a complementary effect on each other.

In May of 1992, University of California, Los Angeles researchers reported on a huge study of 11,000 Americans. They found that increasing intake of vitamin C nearly halved the death rate from heart disease and lengthens life expectancy by up to six years.

More good news is that vitamin C is safe even at high levels of intake. When Linus Pauling began his vitamin C revolution, he was advocating 5,000 to 10,000 mg a day. These recommendations caused scientists to conduct numerous studies on the safety of vitamin C. The literature supports the safety of 5,000 to 10,000 mg a day.

BETA-CAROTENE CUTS HEART PROBLEMS BY HALF

That was the title of an article on beta-carotene which is a form of pro-vitamin A. It is the nutrient that gives deep colored vegetables and fruits their distinctive hues.

The result of this on-going study was reported in the Medical Tribune. A total of 22,000 men were split into two groups. One group took 50 mg (83,000 IU) of beta-carotene every other day and the other group a placebo. At the end of six years, the beta-carotene group had half as many "major cardiovascular events" such as heart attack or stroke. Half of these men were also taking aspirin. It is from this study that the idea originated to give aspirin to heart risk patients.

Beta-carotene could help slow the progress of heart disease. For instance, in one study, 333 men had signs of heart disease, stable angina, bypass surgery or angioplasty. None of the 333 men who took beta-carotene and aspirin had a heart attack. Do they work together? If you want to try the aspirin, discuss it with your physician first.

Beta-carotene is another one of those safe nutrients to take. If you took a lot, your skin would turn an orange color; that's the only side effect. The major studies all seem to focus on an average of 80,000 IU every other day. That would mean five cups of spinach, or two cups of carrots, or 25 cups of broccoli. I like all of these vegetables, but just not that much. I definitely choose to add a beta-carotene food supplement.

B COMPLEX

There are eight members of the B complex, all of which work together like a family. Each helps the other do a better job. Much of the B complex is very fragile and can be destroyed by storage, shipping and cooking. The big three killers of the complex are heat, air and light. For instance, prolonged heating can destroy up to 40 percent of the thiamin in a serving of green beans.

Various members of the B complex have been shown to lower blood cholesterol, lower triglycerides, increase the good HDLs, and expand or widen the blood vessels. Granted, these effects are very small in most cases, but I want all the help I can get. However, some members of the B complex, such a folic acid, offer some really significant heart disease protection. Folic acid is extremely vital in preventing heart disease. A by-product of metabolism called homocysteine can build up in the body and increase the risk of heart disease. The New England Journal of Medicine reported that people with high levels of homocysteine were 30 times more likely to develop vascular disease than those with normal levels.

To put these numbers in perspective, high homocysteine is a more potent risk factor than high cholesterol, high blood pressure, or cigarette smoking! Here is the good news: Folic acid can protect us from homocysteine.

Extra B complex is a must for those over 55. As you age, the B complex is not absorbed as efficiently as when you were younger. As a result, you require a greater concentration of B's for better absorption.

Always add the entire B complex even if you are after the beneficial effects of just one member such as folic acid. Remember, the B complex works as a team, each helping and balancing the other.

CALCIUM

If you decide to become a vegetarian, all of the familiar sources of calcium are eliminated. On the food plan suggested, you are going to be reducing dairy products to only those with a low-fat content.

Some people complain of the somewhat "flat" taste of low-and-non-fat-dairy. Others (some 26 percent) cannot tolerate the lactose in many dairy products. We need over 1,000 mg of calcium, but the sad truth is Americans only average about 660 mg. All this tells me that nearly all Americans need a calcium supplement for optimal health.

Calcium excretion via the bowel has been shown to be beneficial to our heart. We know how soluble fiber binds cholesterol and takes it to elimination; well, calcium gives us more help here. It combines with cholesterol and other fats such as triglycerides and forms soap-like compounds. The body cannot reabsorb these compounds, so they are excreted.

Calcium has also been shown to help lower blood pressure in about 26 percent of those with the problem. This is about the same percentage of people who are sodium sensitive, so there may be some connection.

LECITHIN

Lecithin is a nutrient found in plant and animal tissues. It is mainly produced commercially from soya beans.

Lecithin is a phosphorus lipid made up of choline and inositol, a major component of cell membranes, which regulate the entry and exit of nutrients from the cell.

Lecithin is useful in moving cholesterol out of the body and maintaining a healthy liver. Lecithin does its work of removing cholesterol from the blood through an enzyme called LCAT (lecithin acetyl transferase) that dissolves the accumulated cholesterol and moves it to the liver. Once cholesterol is taken to the liver, it is used for the production of bile.

A 16-week study at Rutgers Medical School showed a "marked decrease in serum cholesterol." A Belgian study with some 100 patients showed a 40 percent drop in cholesterol. In both of those studies, the cholesterol was high to begin with.

Key #5

Include
Cholesterol-Lowering Herbs

There are many herbs that are available to a herbalist to lower your cholesterol and triglycerides. I will just recommend a short list of well-researched herbs.

HAWTHORN

Hawthorn berry extract is an old herbal remedy for heart condition. Herbalist considers this herb as a "heart tonic."

Recent research shows that oxidized LDL cholesterol and not just LDL cholesterol is a villain that causes clogged arteries and heart attacks.

Hawthorn helps reduce cholesterol in the following ways:

- It contains a powerful antioxidant "oligometric proanthocynidins," that helps prevent oxidization of LDL cholesterol in the blood. This process prevents the building up of plaque on the arterial wall (atherosclerosis).

- It helps promote the conversion of LDL cholesterol into HDL (good) cholesterol (Rister R., Japanese Herbal Medicine, Avery 1999, p. 60).

- It prevents cholesterol from accumulating in the liver by encouraging production of cholesterol-laden bile, which passes into the intestine and out of the body.

GUGULIPID (Commiphora mukul)

Gugulipid is a patented extract of gugul (mukul myrrh tree), containing 2.5 percent guggulsterones, its active compound. The word gugul means "gummy resins." It is an Indian Ayurvedic medicine that has a history of at least 3,000 years.

In both human and animal studies, gugulipid helps lower Total cholesterol, LDL and triglycerides and raise HDL cholesterol, although most studies are small.

Research shows that it acts as an anticoagulant by inhibiting blood platelets from clumping together and therefore offers protection against blood clots.

In the United States, a similar story is told. "Significant cholesterol and triglycerides reduction," says Richard Conaut, author of *Natural Alternatives for Lowering Cholesterol and Triglycerides.*

If you are on cholesterol-lowering drugs,

please consult your doctor before taking gugulipid.

Research shows that it is non-toxic and safe to take. In rare cases, gugulipid has been known to cause minor gastrointestinal problems including nausea and gas. Pregnant women should avoid this herb.

TURMERIC

Tumeric is used as a spice especially in India and China. The curcumin in tumeric gives it its orange yellow color.

Curcumin is most noted for its antioxidant, anti-cancer and anti-inflammatory properties. As an anti-inflammatory, turmeric is heart-protective. Many researchers believe that inflammation in the circulating blood plays an important role in triggering heart attacks.

Studies in rabbits and rats fed on a high fat diet have consistently shown that turmeric helps lower LDL cholesterol levels and triglycerides, as well as preventing LDL from being oxidized. However, there are very few studies performed on humans. Since it does work in other animals, it may also work in humans.

Some researchers think that the cholesterol-lowering effect of turmeric might be related to its decreased cholesterol uptake in the intestines and increased production of bile acids in the liver.

Key #6

Take Drugs If Need Be

If healthy lifestyle and nutrition cannot help you lower your cholesterol to a healthy level, drugs may be needed. However, you must continue to practice healthy living along with a proper diet and nutrition as discussed earlier.

Here is one advice, from Dr Alan Beckles of Beth Israel Medical Center, New York, you need to heed before embarking on a drug program. He says, I quote, "The decision for drug therapy is a serious one. All of the drugs on to-day's market to lower serum cholesterol have side effects. There is not one drug that is more free of side effects than another. The decision for drug therapy should be made knowing that the result is clearly beneficial to the patient and vastly outweighs the risk."

Experts now recommend that drug treatments be tailored for raising or lowering specific lipids, depending on the patient's blood lipid picture.

Here are some guidelines from AHA on when to start a drug therapy:

LDL Cholesterol	Level for Drug Consideration (after therapeutic life changes)	Goal of Therapy
Without coronary heart disease and with fewer than two risk factors†	4.9 mmol//L or higher*	Less than 4.1 mmol/L
Without coronary heart disease and with two or more risk factors	4.1 mmol/L or higher	Less than 3.36 mmol/L
With coronary heart disease	3.36mmol/L or higher**	2.58 mmol/L or less

Controlling Cholesterol with Medication

Generally, there are now five major groups of cholesterol-lowering drugs in use:

- Statins (HMG CoA reductase)
- Resins (bile acid sequestrants)
- Fibrates (fibric acid derivatives)
- Niacin (nicotinic acid)
- Cholesterol Absorption Inhibitors

Your doctor will be the best person to advise you on which cholesterol-lowering drug or in combination would be suitable for you. Under no circumstances should you embark on drugs to help you lower your cholesterol without your doctor's approval.

Below, briefly is a bird's eye view of the drugs currently available to treat diabetes. I repeat, your doctor is the only one qualified to prescribe drugs to lower your cholesterol.

STATINS

Many doctors prescribe statins as the first choice to lower LDL cholesterol. They work by blocking an enzyme called HMG-CoA reductase which controls the rate of cholesterol production in the liver.

Statins can lower cholesterol 20-60 percent by slowing the production of cholesterol and by increasing the liver's ability to remove LDL already in the blood. They have a modest effect on triglycerides and give a mild boost to your HDL cholesterol.

Statins come in tablets or capsules and are usually taken with the evening meal or at bedtime.

Well known brand of statins include: Lipitor, Zocor, Altoprev, Crestor, Lescol, Mevacor and Pravachol.

Cautions and Possible Side Effects:
Statin drugs go down well with most people, however, they do have some negative side effects. Side effects include: Constipation, nausea, diarrhea, stomach pain, cramps, muscle soreness, pain and weakness.

Damage to the liver is the most serious side effect of statins. If you are on statins, your doctor will recommend periodic tests to monitor the effect of the medication on your liver. If you have elevated liver enzyme or a history of liver disease or you are pregnant, avoid taking statins.

Studies have shown that statin drugs disrupt

the body's ability to produce Coenzyme Q10, which helps the body cells convert food into energy. In many countries CoQ10 is prescribed to treat congestive heart failure. Supplement your diet with CoQ10 if you are on statins.

BILE ACID SEQUESTRANTS (RESINS)

This class of LDL-lowering drugs works by binding bile acids in the intestine and disposing them out of the body. Bile acids help with the absorption of dietary fat and cholesterol.

This is how it works. Your body makes bile from cholesterol and if the bile acids are being removed by this class of drugs, your liver responds by making more bile needed to break down fatty foods. In order to produce more bile acids, the liver converts more cholesterol into bile acids, which lowers the level of cholesterol in the blood.

Besides lowering LDL cholesterol, it improves HDL moderately but may raise your triglycerides. So people with triglycerides levels higher than 3.0 mmol/L should opt for another class of drugs.

Bile acid sequestrants are poorly tolerated at high doses but when used in low doses in combination with statins along with dietary therapy; they are shown to lower LDL cholesterol by as much as 50 percent.

Side Effects
This class of drugs can cause gastrointestinal

discomfort such as bloating, constipation, weight loss, vomiting, abdominal pain, diarrhea, and flatulence.

They also reduce the absorption of vitamins A, D, E and K. If a patient is on long-term therapy it could cause a deficiency in these vitamins.

You should avoid this class of drugs if your triglyceride levels are above 7.7 mmol/L or 300 mg/dL, or you are experiencing a bad bout of constipation.

Brands available include: Questran, Colestid and WelChol.

FIBRATES (FIBRIC ACID DERIVATIVES)

Fibrates are best used to reduce triglycerides and in patients who cannot tolerate statins. They have little impact on your HDL and LDL cholesterol.

They were widely used before the statins arrived. They probably act by inhibiting lipoprotein lipase activity which results in a triglyceride-lowering effect. Gemfibrozil is the fibrate most widely used in the United States.

Fibrates are generally well tolerated by most patients. Gastrointestinal discomfort is the most common side effect. Fibrates may increase the likelihood of developing cholesterol gallstones. Fibrates can also increase the effect of medications that thin the blood when the doses are given far above the recommended dosage.

As a result, it is used less often than other

drugs in patients with heart disease. Brands available include Lopid, Tricor and Atromid-S.

NIACIN

Niacin (vitamin B3) is the first choice of patients with low HDL levels. Niacin lowers LDL cholesterol and triglycerides and raises HDL cholesterol. It is one of the oldest cholesterol-reducing agents around with a long-standing track record of effectiveness and safety.

Niacin comes in prescription form and as food supplements. Dietary supplement niacin must *not* be used as a substitute for prescription niacin. Doses above 1500 milligrams per day should be taken only on consultation with your doctor.

Side Effects

Niacin side effects include flushing, itching, stomach upset, gout and elevate liver enzymes. Diabetic should use niacin with caution as it can raise blood sugar levels. In spite of these drawbacks, it is still one of the oldest cholesterol-reducing agents around with a long-standing track record of effectiveness and safety.

Popular brands include: Niaspan, Nicolar and Slo-Niacin.

CHOLESTEROL ABSORPTION INHIBITORS (Zetia)

The generic name for Zetia is Ezetimibe. It was approved by the US Food and Drug Administration

(FDA) in late 2002. This class of drugs is commonly prescribed as a cholesterol absorption inhibitor to lower levels of LDL cholesterol. It mildly reduces triglycerides.

This drug works in the digestive tract by reducing the amount of cholesterol absorbed from foods you eat. It is important that you stay on a cholesterol-lowering diet plan while taking this medicine.

Zetia is taken once daily, with or without food. Try to take Zetia at the same time each day. Zetia is most useful in people who cannot take statin drugs for one reason or another.

Side Effects
The most common reported side effects of Zetia include stomach pain and tiredness, diarrhea, back pain, joint pain, and sinusitis. Avoid this medication if you are allergic to Zetia or if you have liver disease.

WORK WITH YOUR DOCTOR

Tell your doctor right away if you have any side effects. Do not stop taking your medicine unless your doctor tells you to.

Key #7

Start Loving Your Heart Now

To win the cholesterol war, you must commit to live a healthy lifestyle and eat right before resorting to drugs. Many people give up on healthy eating because their diet is based on their taste buds. Don't be like these people. If you love your life, start loving your heart.

Do not wait for symptoms to appear. In 50 percent of deaths from a heart attack, sudden death was the very first symptom! Solid research reports that for each one percent reduction in blood cholesterol, you decrease your chances of a heart attack by an amazing two percent! Some studies are even indicating the reduction may approach three percent.

Prevention is the only way the epidemic of heart disease can be arrested. We have the knowledge for prevention and we have the knowledge to prevent a tremendous amount of death, disability, and suffering right now if we are wise enough to apply it. This is what I want to share with you in this book.

There is no longer any excuse for tolerating heart attack risk factors that are *under your control*. There are few people, very few, who have a genetic predisposition for higher cholesterol.

Here is the challenge. Have your blood lipid profile taken as we talked about in Key #1. This involves the total analysis of the fats in your blood including Total cholesterol, HDL cholesterol, LDL cholesterol, triglycerides, and some others. From these figures, you can compute some of the ratios I mentioned in Key #1. Know your numbers! Are you headed for a heart attack – or will you escape?

After that, start the plan I recommend. Follow the simple plan I recommended religiously for four to six weeks. Then have another blood lipid profile done.

That's all there is to it! At the end of four to six weeks your cholesterol will have dropped by at least 10 percent. That means, if you began at 6.2, you should be at least down to 5.59 by the end of the challenge time. Stick with the program, and your blood lipid profile should continue to improve and you decrease your heart attack risk.

In some people it drops much more, depending on how high it was at the start. Even more importantly, some other risk factors will improve significantly. The various ratios of lipids, many of which are now considered more important than Total cholesterol, will greatly improve. You will have reduced your chances of a heart attack dramatically!

Once you have a little success under your belt, keep to the program until you achieve the optimal numbers I have referred to in the book. Then, you will be on the way to adding years to your life and life to your years.

Bibliography

Agarwal RC, et al. "Clinical trial of gugulipid – a new hypolipidemic agent of plant origin in primary hyperlipidemia." *Indian J. Med. Res.* 1986 Dec; 84: 626-34.

Ascherio A, et al. "Trans-fatty acids intake and risk of myocardial infarction." *Circulation.* 1994; 89:94-101.

Ames B. "Oxidants, antioxidants, and degenerative diseases of aging." Proceedings of National Academy of Sciences, 90(17): 7915-22, 1993.

Anderson, D. M., Castelli, W. P. and Levy, D. "Cholesterol and mortality: 30 years of follow-up from the Framingham Study." *Journal of the American Medical Association,* 257: 2176-80, 1987.

Behall KM, et al. "Effect of beta-glucan level in oat fiber extracts on blood lipids in men and women." *J Am Coll Nutr.* 1997; 16: 46-51.

Bell S, Goldman, et al. "Effect of beta-glucan from oats and yeast on serum lipids." *Crit Rev Food Sci Nutr.* 1999; 39: 189-202.

Best MM, et al. "Lowering of serum cholesterol by the administration of a plant sterol." *Circulation* 1954; 10: 201-6.

Blair SN, et al. "Incremental reduction of serum Total cholesterol and low-density lipoprotein cholesterol with the addition of plant stanol ester-containing spread to statin therapy." *Am J Cardiol.* 2000; 86: 46-52.

Braaten JT, et al. "Oat beta-glucan reduces blood cholesterol concentration in hypercholesterolemic subjects." *Eur J*

Clin Nutr. 1994; 48: 465-474.

Brody J. Jane Brody's "Good Food Book." Bantam Books 1987.

Caroll, K. "Review of clinical studies on cholesterol-lowering response to soy protein." *Journal of the American Dietetic Association,* 91: 820-87, 1991.

Carper, J. "The Good Pharmacy Guide to Good Eating." Bantam Books 1991.

Cooper, K. "The Aerobics Program for Total Well-Being." Bantam Books, 1982. Also, Cooper K. and Cooper, M. "The New Aerobics for Women." Rev. ed. Bantam Books, 1988.

Dwyer, J. T. "Health aspects of vegetarian diets." *American Journal of Clinical Nutrition,* 48 (3 suppl.): 712-38, 1988.

Food and Drug Administration, HHS. "Food labeling: Health claims; soluble dietary fiber from certain foods and coronary heart disease." Final rule. *Fed Regist.* 2003; 68: 44207-44209.

Gaziano, J. "The role of beta-carotene in the prevention of cardiovascular disease." Annals of the New York Academy of Sciences, 691: 148-55. 1993.

Grundy SM. "Stanol esters as dietary adjunct to cholesterol-lowering therapies." *Eur Heart J* 1999; 1: S132-S138.

Griffin, et al. "How To Lower Your Cholesterol and Beat the Odds of a Heart Attack." Fisher Books, 1993.

Gylling H, Miettinen TA. "Cholesterol

reduction by different plant stanol mixtures and with variable fat intake." *Metabolism.* 1999; 48: 575-580.

Haskell, W et al. "The role of water-soluble dietary fiber in the management of elevated plasma cholesterol in healthy subjects." *American Journal of Cardiology,* 69: 433-9, 1992.

Hobbs, C., Foster S. "Hawthorn: A Literature Review." *Herbalgram* 1990; 22: 19-33.

Hoffman, R. "Antioxidants and the prevention of coronary heart disease." Archives of Internal Medicines, 155(3): 241-46, 1995.

Jacques, P. "Effects of vitamin C on high density lipoprotein, cholesterol and blood pressure." *Journal of the American College of Nutrition,* 62: 252-55, 1992.

Jensen, C., Spiller, et al. "The effect of acacia gum and water-soluble dietary fiber mixture on blood lipids in humans." *Journal of the American College of Nutrition,* 12:147-54, 1993.

Jialal, I. "The effect of a-tocopherol supplementation on LDL oxidation and vitamin E: A dose response study." *Atherosclerosis, Thrombosis and Vascular Biology,* 15(2): 190-198, 1995.

Katan MB, Zock PL, Mensink RP. "Trans fatty acids and their effects on lipoproteins in humans." *Annual Review of Nutrition.* 1995; 15: 473-93.

Lands, W. "Biochemistry and physiology of n-3 fatty acids." *FASEB Journal,* 6: 2530-36, 1992.

Law M. "Plant sterol and stanol margarines and health." *BMJ,* 2000; 320: 861-864.

Lees AM, et al. "Plant sterols as cholesterol-lowering agents: Clinical trials in patients with hyper-cholesterolemia and studies of sterol balance." *Atherosclerosis* 1977; 28: 325-38.

Manson, J. "Antioxidants and cardiovascular disease: a review." *Journal of the American College of Nutrition,* 12(4): 426-32, August 1993.

Miettinen TA, et al. "Reduction of serum cholesterol with sitostanol-ester margarine in a mildly hyper-cholesterolemic population." *N Engl J Med* 1995; 333: 1308-12.

Mindell, E. "Earl Mindell's Soy Miracle." Fireside. 1995.

Nguyen TT. "The cholesterol-lowering action of plant stanol esters." *J Nutr.* 1999; 129: 2109-2112.

Niaz, MA, and Chosh, S. "Hypolipidemic and antioxidant effects of Commiphora mukul (gugulipid) as an adjunct to dietary therapy in patients with hypercholesterolmia." *Cardiovascular Drugs and Therapeutics* (1994) 8: 659-664.

Nityanand S. et al. "Clinical Trials with gugulipid. A new Hypolipidemic Agent." *J Assoc. Physicians India* 37: 5 (May 1989): 323-28.

Plat J, van Onselen EN, van Heugten MM, et al. "Effects on serum lipids, lipoproteins and fat soluble antioxidant concentrations of consumption frequency of margarines and shortenings enriched with plant stanol esters." *Eur J Clin Nutr.* 2000; 54: 671-677.

Plat J, Mensink RP. "Plant stanol and sterol esters in the control of blood cholesterol levels: Mechanism and safety aspects." *Am Journal of Cardiology,* 2005 Jul 4; 96 (1A): 15D.

"Pressing garlic for possible health benefits." Tufts University Diet and Nutrition Letter, 12(7): 3, September 1994.

Sacks, F. "Therapy to molecular mechanisms." *Annals of the New York Academy of Sciences* 676: 188-201, 1993.

Slavin, J. "Nutrition benefits of soy protein and soy fiber." Journal of the American Dietetic Association, 91: 816-19, 1991.

Stampfer, M. "Homocysteine and marginal vitamin deficiency: The importance of adequate vitamin intake." Editorial. *Journal of the American Medical Association,* 270(22): 2726, 1993.

Stampfer M. "Vitamin E consumption and the risk of coronary disease in women." *New England Journal of Medicine,* 328: 1444-49, 1993.

Street D. "Serum antioxidants and myocardial infarction." *Circulation,* 90: 1154-19, 1994.

"Third Report of the NCEP Expert Panel on Detection, Evaluation, and Treatment of High Blood Cholesterol in Adults, also known as Adult Treatment Panel (ATP) III." *Journal of the American Medical Association* May 16, 2001.

Thomas T. and Londeree, B. "Energy cost during prolonged walking vs. jogging exercise." *The Physician and Sports Medicine* 17: 93-102, 1989.

Uusitupa MI, Ruuskanen E, Makinen E, et al. "A controlled study on the effect of beta-glucan-rich oat bran on serum lipids in hypercholesterolemic subjects: Relation to apolipoprotein E phenotype." *J Am Coll Nutr.* 1992; 11: 651-659.

"Vegetarian – live longer." *British Medical Journal,* 308: 1667-771, 1994.

Willett WC, Stampfer MJ, Manson JE, et al. "Intake of trans fatty acids and risk of coronary heart disease among women." *Lancet,* 1993; 341: 581-5.

Zawistowski J. "A functional ingredient for maintaining cardiovascular health: phytosterols." Presented at Functional Foods and Beverages Forum; 2004 Oct 27; Orlando.

Glossary

Aerobic exercise: It is anything that makes you breathe a bit more heavily and increases the pulse rate.

Angina: A condition in which the heart muscles receive an insufficient blood supply, resulting in chest pain in the left arm and shoulder. The chest pain of angina is typically severe and crushing.

Artery: A large blood vessel that carries blood from the heart to other parts of the body. Arteries are thicker and have walls that are stronger and more elastic than the walls of veins.

Atherosclerosis: A process of progressive clogging, narrowing and hardening of the walls of the body's large arteries and medium-sized blood vessels as a result of fat deposits on their inner lining. Atherosclerosis is the root cause of most cardiovascular disease.

Beta-glucan: It is a soluble fiber found in the cell walls of grains particularly from oats and barley. In the body it transforms into a sticky gel that coats the intestine. Here the beta-glucan targets the LDL faction and dietary fat and flushes them out of the body.

Bile Acid Sequestrants: This class of LDL lowering drugs works by binding bile acids in the intestine and disposing them out of the body

Blood vessels: Tubes that carry blood to and from all parts of the body. The three main types of blood vessels are arteries, veins, and capillaries.

Body Mass Index (BMI): A measure used to evaluate body weight relative to a person's height. BMI is used to find out if a person is underweight, normal weight, overweight or obese. To calculate your BMI, divide your weight by your height squared.

Cardiovascular disease: Disease of the heart and blood vessels (arteries, veins, and capillaries).

Cholesterol: An odorless, white, powdery fatty substance similar to fat produced by the liver and found in the blood. It is also found in some foods. Cholesterol is used by the body to make hormones and build cell walls. An elevated level of blood cholesterol is a major cause of coronary heart disease.

Cholesterol Absorption Inhibitors (Zetia): This class of drugs is commonly prescribed as a cholesterol absorption inhibitor to lower levels of LDL cholesterol. It mildly reduces triglycerides.

Congestive heart failure: Loss of the heart's pumping power, which causes fluids to collect in the body, especially in the feet and lungs. Congestive heart failure often develops gradually over several years, although it also can happen suddenly.

Coronary heart disease: This disease is caused by narrowing of the arteries that supply blood to the heart mainly due to cholesterol deposits in the artery walls. If the blood supply is cut off, the result is a heart attack.

Diabetes: Diabetes results when our body cannot use blood glucose as energy because of having too little insulin or being unable to use insulin. There are two major forms of diabetes. In type 1 diabetes the pancreas no longer makes insulin and therefore blood glucose cannot enter the cells to be used for energy. In type 2 diabetes, either the pancreas does not make enough insulin or the body is unable to use insulin correctly.

Fibrates: They are a class of drugs best used to reduce triglycerides and in patients who cannot tolerate statins.

Free radicals: Are incomplete,

unstable molecules which are basic building blocks in nature such as oxygen, fatty acids and amino acids.

Glucose: Glucose is the principal sugar the body makes. It is the body's main source of energy. The body makes glucose from proteins, fats and carbohydrates. Glucose is carried to each cell through the bloodstream.

Gugulipid: Is a patented extract of gugul (mukul myrrh tree) that helps lower Total Cholesterol, LDL and triglycerides and raise HDL cholesterol.

Hawthorn: It is a berry extract from the hawthorn shrub with thorny branches. It contains a powerful antioxidant "oligometric proanthocynidins" that helps prevent oxidization of LDL cholesterol in the blood. Herbalists call it a "heart tonic."

HDL cholesterol: High-density lipoprotein (HDL), the "good" cholesterol found in the blood that takes extra cholesterol from the bloodstream to the liver for removal.

Heart attack: A heart attack occurs from the blockage in one of the coronary arteries due to atherosclerosis. The blockage stops the blood supply to the heart muscle. Without the necessary oxygen that comes in the blood, the part affected becomes damaged. Depending upon the severity of the damage, disability or death can result.

Hyperlipidemia: Higher than normal fat and cholesterol levels in the blood.

Insulin: A natural hormone made by the pancreas that controls the level of the sugar glucose in the blood. Insulin permits cells to use glucose for energy. Cells cannot utilize glucose without insulin.

Insulin resistance: A condition in which the body cells refuse to let insulin shuttle glucose into it. This resistance by the cells causes glucose to remain high in the bloodstream.

LDL cholesterol: Low-density lipoprotein (LDL), a fat found in the blood, takes cholesterol around the body to where it is needed for cell repair and also deposits it on the inside of artery walls. It is often called "bad" cholesterol.

Lipid: A term for fat in the body. Lipids can be broken down by the body and used for energy.

Lipoprotein: These are proteins that act like trucks, picking up the cholesterol and transporting it to different parts of the body.

Lipoproteins are either high-density or low-density, based on how much protein and fat they have. The lower the density of the lipoprotein, the more fats it contains.

Mg/dL: Milligrams per deciliter. The units used by Americans when measuring blood glucose and lipid levels. European countries use SI units (mmol/L).

Niacin: This class of drugs lowers LDL cholesterol and triglycerides and raises HDL cholesterol.

Omega-3 fatty acids: Also known as polyunsaturated fatty acids are essential fatty acids. They are essential to human health but cannot be manufactured by the body and must be obtained from food. Omega-3 fatty acids can be found in fish such as salmon, tuna and halibut, and other marine life such as algae and nut oils. There are three major types of omega-3 fatty acids that are ingested in foods and used by the body: Alpha-linolenic acid (ALA), eicosapentaenoic acid (EPA), and docosahexaenoic acid (DHA).

Phytochemicals: Are non-nutritive plant chemicals that have protective or disease preventive properties. Lycopene in tomatoes, isoflavones in soy and flavanoids in fruits are some common examples.

Psyllium Seed husk: It is a potent natural soluble fiber from the husk of the psyllium seed of the Plantago ovata plant. It has the support of the U.S Food and Drug Administration to be used in food and supplements to help people to maintain healthy cholesterol and blood lipid profile.

Saturated fats: Have high melting points and are usually solid at room temperature. Eating excessive saturated fats can increase cholesterol in your blood more than consuming cholesterol!

Stanols: They are *saturated components* of vegetable oils and plants. Like the sterols, they have also cholesterol lowering properties.

Statins: This class of drugs is the first choice of many doctors to prescribe to lower LDL cholesterol. They work by blocking an enzyme called HMG-CoA reductase to control the rate of cholesterol production in the liver.

Sterols: They are *unsaturated components* of vegetable oils and fats and it has powerful cholesterol lowering properties. Sterols of plants are called phytosterols. There are over 60 types of plant sterols but the most common form is beta-sitosterol.

Stroke: The death of brain cells due to a lack of oxygen when the blood flow to the brain is impaired by blockage or rupture of an artery to the brain. This may cause loss of ability to speak or to move parts of the body.

Trans fat: This is created during a process called hydrogenation when food manufacturers add heat, pressure and hydrogen gas to unsaturated vegetable oils to turn it into solid or semi-solid fat. The last 15 years of nutrition research has shown that this "man-made fat" is worse than saturated fat for your heart health.

Triglyceride: The storage form of fat in the body. High triglyceride levels may occur when diabetes is out of control.

Vein: A blood vessel that carries blood to the heart.

Waist circumference measurement: This is a measurement of abdominal fat.

Waist-to-hip ratio: Refers to the comparison of weight carried between your waist and hips. It is a simple measure of where your fats are distributed in your body.

Simple books for understanding health

 OAK BETTER HEALTH SERIES

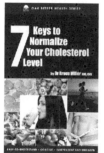

7 Keys to Normalize Your Cholesterol Level
In this book, you will discover seven keys in simple and concise language, you can take to lower your cholesterol to a healthy level.

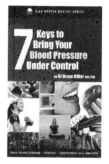

7 Keys To Bring Your Blood Pressure Under Control
This book gives you seven crucial keys you can take today to lower your blood pressure and keep it under control or prevent it in the first place. Start using these keys today to avoid becoming a candidate for a heart attack or stroke.

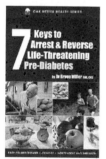

7 Keys to Arrest & Reverse Life-Threatening Pre-Diabetes
This book lays down seven keys to avoid being a victim of full blown diabetes. This will add years to your life and life to your years as pre-diabetes causes heart attack or stroke, two main silent killers of the human race.

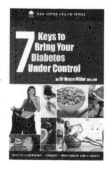

7 Keys to Bring Your Diabetes Under Control
Within these easy-to-read pages, you will find seven crucial keys to help you control your sugar level to near normal as possible and improve your cell's sensitivity to insulin to prevent or delay the onset of long-term complications of the disease.